C000228795

'This book was written by a practitioner steeped i
It offers invaluable insight to professionals work
as residential units or schools. It is recommended
practitioners and those starting to navigate their w
and its aftermath.'

Graham Music, *PhD, consultant child and adolescent psychotherapist,*
Tavistock Centre, author of Nurturing Natures *and* Nurturing Children

'Building on the pioneering work of Winnicott and her own professional experience,
Bradley has integrated recent findings to produce a model of practice which offers
structure whilst fostering spontaneity and creativity. This framework makes a
valuable contribution, enabling practitioners to build a deeper understanding of
the children in their care and provide them with the individualised therapeutic care
they need to recover from profound early trauma.'

Adrian Sutton, *MB BS, FRC Psych., professor, director,*
Squiggle Foundation, Hon Senior Lecturer in Medical Education,
University of Manchester

'Early trauma too often results in lives that are overwhelmed by the challenge of
managing life itself. It can lead to life-long destructive behaviour and – as I have
seen too often in my work with prisoners – condemns damaged young people to a
criminal justice system ill-equipped to do anything but add to their profound and
enduring sense of dislocation. There is a better answer, a life-changing answer –
effective, proven, therapeutic intervention. This important and urgent book should
be required reading for all involved in policy-making and funding decisions around
young people, setting out clearly and persuasively what can be done is based on
Christine Bradley's four decades of working in the field and the extraordinary
results that follow.'

Peter Stanford, *writer, editor, and director,*
the Longford Trust for Prison Reform

Trauma in Children and Young People

This book offers a unique combination of an in-depth examination of attachment, a refined and tested model of Needs Led Assessment and Therapeutic Treatment Plans, and applies it to specific contexts including those of children in residential/ foster care, young offenders, and unaccompanied asylum-seeking minors.

Trauma in Children and Young People, the culmination of 40 years of experience in the field, focuses on the lives of children and young people who have experienced and lived with the repercussion of early trauma. Accompanied with case studies, it examines how therapeutic intervention can enable children and young people to connect with their inner world of fragmented feelings and emotions and to develop a sense of 'self' that is real and has meaning.

This book is intended for professionals working therapeutically with traumatised children, such as therapists, psychologists, psychiatrists, mental health workers, social pedagogues, child and youth care workers, social workers, residential care workers and foster carers, teachers, youth justice workers, and child refugee agencies.

Christine Bradley has worked with vulnerable children for over 40 years. Her career began as a therapeutic resource worker at the Cotswold Community and Mulberry Bush School in the 1970s and 80s, both pioneering therapeutic communities for children and young people during that period. She is a consultant psychotherapist for organisations in residential care, therapeutic communities, and adoption/fostering agencies and a fellow of Dartington Social Policy Research Unit. Christine Bradley was previously a senior officer for LB of Wandsworth and director of the Caldecott College in Kent and has lectured widely, including in Australia and Europe.

Francia Kinchington, MA Ed. Psych. SFHEA, MBPsS, is an education consultant, analyst, and editor with publications and expertise in leadership, psychology, change, and development in Higher Education and in schools, both internationally and in the UK. Formally a principal lecturer at the University of Greenwich for 25 years, she is an experienced doctoral supervisor and examiner, with 25 doctoral completions. She is a graduate member of the British Psychological Society and senior fellow of the Higher Education Academy.

Trauma in Children and Young People

Reaching the Heart of the Matter

Christine Bradley
with Francia Kinchington

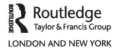

Routledge
Taylor & Francis Group

LONDON AND NEW YORK

Designed cover image: © Kind permission for use of the cover
image has been authorised by Maple House Residential Children's
Home

First published 2024
by Routledge
4 Park Square, Milton Park, Abingdon, Oxon OX14 4RN

and by Routledge
605 Third Avenue, New York, NY 10158

Routledge is an imprint of the Taylor & Francis Group, an informa business

© 2024 Christine Bradley with Francia Kinchington

British Library Cataloguing-in-Publication Data
A catalogue record for this book is available from the British Library

Library of Congress Cataloging-in-Publication Data
Names: Bradley, Christine (Christine Mary), 1945- author. | Kinchington,
Francia, author.
Title: Trauma in children and young people : reaching the heart of the
matter / Christine Bradley with Francia Kinchington.
Description: Abingdon, Oxon ; New York, NY : Routledge, 2024. | Includes
bibliographical references and index. |
Identifiers: LCCN 2023006537 (print) | LCCN 2023006538 (ebook) |
ISBN 9780367678029 (hbk.) | ISBN 9780367678005 (pbk) | ISBN
9781003132882 (ebk)
Subjects: LCSH: Psychic trauma in children—Treatment. | Psychic trauma
in adolescence—Treatment. | Post-traumatic stress disorder in children—
Treatment. | Child abuse—Treatment. | Abused children—Rehabilitaiton.
Classification: LCC RJ506.P66 B73 2024 (print) | LCC RJ506.P66 (ebook) |
DDC 618.92/8521—dc23/eng/20230607
LC record available at https://lccn.loc.gov/2023006537
LC ebook record available at https://lccn.loc.gov/2023006538

ISBN: 9780367678029 (hbk)
ISBN: 9780367678005 (pbk)
ISBN: 9781003132882 (ebk)

DOI: 10.4324/9781003132882

Typeset in Times New Roman
by codeMantra

Contents

Acknowledgements

There are many people that we wish to thank for the support and kindness that they have given during the writing of this book:

All the young people who have allowed their stories to be told
The Tunstall Jubilee Foundation for funding
Judith Trowell for her ongoing support and analytic guidance
Dominic from Williams Computers for his ongoing support

For their time and help in providing information for the chapters:
Caroline Shaw and her team at Ashford Day Nursery
Cian Hughes and his team at Kingfisher View, My Choice Children's Organisation
Carly Thomas and her team at Willow Trees, Caldecott Foundation
Elaine Rose and Sam Barling from Kent Adoption
Ray Ashton and his team at Lake House, Channels and Choices
Sarah Whiting and her foster team at Channels and Choices
Chris Martin and his team at Maple House, My Choice Children's Organisation
Lilian Simonson and her team at Enthum
Sheila Melzak and her team at the Baobab Centre for Young Survivors in Exile
Razia and Gareth with their team at Kent Refugee Action Group
Celia Sadie for her insight on young offenders

For reading chapters:
Brian Bishop
Annie Bousfield
John Clegg
Geoff Gildersleeve
Maureen Howard
Sue Norrington
Maureen Rossi
John Whitwell

Foreword

Having experienced childhood trauma, I still search for answers, understanding, and a sense of belonging. As a child I felt my needs were not met in residential care and struggled to be met while I was in foster care. As an adult I can see that it is hard to meet complex needs without appropriate service provision, professional training, and commitment and 'coming into contact with the right people' who cross your path. Communicating my feelings was virtually impossible as a child and something I still feel to some degree now, when speaking about the traumas I faced. Not every emotion, experience, and reaction can always be explained – acceptance and acknowledgement are sometimes more powerful. I had some profoundly positive relationships with professionals while I was in care; however, I experienced many negative ones too.

Reaching the Heart of the Matter is a positive, insightful, and thoughtful account of searching to understand childhood trauma and intervention. While we as a society understand more about traumatic experiences now, there is still so much which is not understood. I felt that there were very few professionals that understood my experiences while in care, though I do feel lucky enough that the very few I had, supported, believed, and did not judge me. I firmly believe that professionals who seek to understand childhood trauma deserve all of the training, funding, and support they need. This will in turn reach all of those children who have suffered and experienced childhood trauma. Christine's dedication and persistent search to understand childhood trauma, professional intervention, and need are very close to my heart.

When society addresses trauma and intervention, a holistic approach needs to be taken. My experience in residential care was an attempt at therapeutic treatment. At the time, and to this day, it felt, and still feels, as though there were not the resources to embed this approach, an approach that I like many others needed. That said, it's important to raise the question about timing and motivation from the perspective of the traumatised child. The resources need to be there and accessible, and critically, these resources and therapeutic input need to be led to some degree by the child. Like adults, children need to address their traumas in their own time. Service provision and therapeutic expertise should be accessible when the timing is right for that individual.

As Christine has pointed out, there are better outcomes in terms of mental health for young people if they have positive experiences with caregivers and therapeutic surroundings. I can definitely relate to this. I had positive and negative experiences from both, and the strength of the positive input stays with me now and is a reminder as to how diverse individual experience can be in the complex 'world' of trauma and the child.

Therapy started for me when I was accepted, not judged, but viewed as an 'individual'. I did not want to be the face of trauma; I wanted to be seen as me, essentially normal and similar to my peers. The individuals that had a therapeutic impact were professionals who liked me for me, wanted to get to know me, were not overly intrigued by my trauma, and were accepting of my feelings. There have always been assumptions of how I feel, but those assumptions created a barrier to me expressing myself. I wanted my feelings to be mine and not generalised feelings around trauma. There isn't a timeline around trauma, but allowing space is an important part of the healing process.

Gayle

Gayle's account of her time in the care system outlines both the positive and negative experiences that she has taken in, experiences which have helped her to achieve a positive outcome in her life. Although some children share this positive experience, unfortunately, we do also need to recognise that for a large number of looked-after children and young people, their experiences were more negative than positive. The starting point for the content of this book is a reminder of the importance of children and young people in need of specialist care and treatment. These young people have been exposed to a continuation of traumatic experiences in their life, which has left them feeling emotionally fragile, often unable to manage the stressful situations they have to face in their life when managing the sometimes difficult and challenging reality in their day-to-day living. Whilst in their placements, it is crucial that these young people experience a sense of believing that the fears and anxieties are being listened to, and taken seriously by those who are responsible for them. Only by delivering such practice will both the child or young person and the workers feel that they are truly reaching the heart of the matter. It is this that will enable the child or young person to develop a more genuine and real sense of self that they can live with and emotionally develop through.

This book covers elements of practice in residential care, fostering, adoption, young offenders, refugee, and asylum-seeking children and young people, outlining that all the young people have experienced traumatic situations in their life which have become unbearable and importantly, that they are unable to think about or resolve. I hope that this book proves that the heart of the matter can be reached by carers, families, specialist workers, and teachers, providing insight and guidance to those responsible for funding and training, and ultimately offering more positive outcomes on behalf of children and young people in need.

Christine Bradley

Introduction

Introduction

The challenge for this book is to understand the impact of the destructive experiences faced by children and young people whose lives have been dominated and shaped by trauma. It is only through this understanding and the insight that it brings that we are able to 'reach the heart of the matter'. In my professional experience over the past 40 years, the task faced by workers in meeting the needs of these young people has become more difficult and complex.

This book is key to the lives of these children and young people; it is about them becoming connected with their inner world of feeling and emotion where their 'self' is real and has meaning. The worker and carer play a critical role, using their knowledge and insight to understand and reflect on the non-explainable behaviour that the young person is unable to think about or work through. This can enable them to work through to a deeper understanding of their own inner world of intense emotions about which they are unable to communicate and unaware of the effect of their behaviours on others. It is not an easy task for workers to evolve their practice and maintain appropriate therapeutic interventions that help children and young people to overcome the impact of their early experiences, to strengthen their sense of self so that they feel more alive and real in their day-to-day lives.

Lives that are defined by mental health issues and an extreme level of emotional deprivation need to be addressed and understood as a matter of urgency. To do this, it is critical that carers and other professionals develop a deeper and more profound insight into how they can provide for and meet the emotional needs of this group of children and young people. It is imperative that the issues and repercussions sur-rounding their experiences are seen and understood not only at a personal level, but at a societal level, both nationally and globally.

The professional role faced by workers and carers in tackling this challenge and working towards helping these children and young people to develop a stronger sense of self so that they become more able to manage the challenges of reality without breakdown occurring is difficult and complex. These workers and carers need to have the insight, understanding, and skills to break through the barriers that lie behind the behaviours and anxieties to reach some of the most unbearable

DOI: 10.4324/9781003132882-1

aspects that have been locked away in the inner world of these children and young people, preventing the development of their thinking, emotional and social growth, and critically their sense of self.

The impact of trauma on the child's emotional maturation can prevent them from becoming an individual who is more able to manage the demands of external reality without breaking down and becoming destructive or self-destructive in their behaviour. Of concern is the rise in mental health problems in children and young people (Newlove-Delgado, 2021:3) where one in six children aged five to 16 were identified as having a probable mental health problem (July 2021), a rise from one in nine in 2017. Further, Simkiss (2012:2) reported that looked-after children and care leavers were more vulnerable, being four and five times more likely to self-harm in adulthood, and carried underlying childhood mental, emotional, behavioural problems and conduct disorders. Of note was that up to half of the young people held in young offender institutions, were, or had previously been in care (Blades *et al.,* 2011:1).

Some 40,000 refugee children and young people arrive in the UK each year. They are strangers in a foreign land, and having come through ordeals of persecution and violence in their own countries, they now find themselves facing what they feel to be the same difficulties. The legacy of this is the creation of more serious mental health difficulties, often resulting in destructive and self-destructive behaviour towards both themselves and others.

Provision for dealing with so many children and young people with the range of problems they present is currently inadequate. So where do we find the starting point in facing these complexities? Much of the current work and effort has focused on reaching a diagnosis for children and young people who display behaviour problems which are difficult and unmanageable. Psychiatric assessment can diagnose a range of syndromes, including attachment disorders, obsessive-compulsive disorder, narcissistic personality, and anti-social behaviour. However, the critical questions that must be asked are, after assessment and diagnosis, what specific treatment and intervention plans have been put in place to address the child's needs? Do the assessment and diagnosis give us a true picture of the inner world of the child or young person? Does it provide their carer with the practical tools to help the child or young person to develop a stronger sense of self, to feel emotionally stronger and acquire the capacity and confidence to manage the outside world without breakdown occurring? A lack of appropriate therapeutic intervention from their workers and carers can result in behaviour which displays impulsive and uncontrollable feelings and inhibited emotions that cannot be thought about or expressed through words. This can result in their behaviour becoming destructive externally, towards others, or self-destructive towards themselves. Often, their placement becomes non-viable and breaks down, and the long-term outcome for the child or young person consequently is negative and debilitating, impacting on their thinking, their sense of being a person with a sense of value, and their level of functioning.

The term childhood trauma used in this book is that used by De Bellis and Zisk (2014:1) derived from the Diagnostic and Statistical Manual of Mental Disorders IV and V (2013), namely,

> exposure to actual or threatened death, serious injury, or sexual violence. This includes experiences of direct trauma exposure, witnessing trauma or learning about trauma that happened to a close friend or relative. In children, motor vehicle accidents, bullying, terrorism, exposure to war, child maltreatment (physical, sexual, and emotional abuse; neglect) and exposure to domestic and community violence.

It is acknowledged that children may experience traumatic events, but the ameliorating factor to the long-term impact of these events is the presence of a supportive and nurturing carer who has the capacity to communicate with the child and understand the child's perception of the experience enabling them to work through it and develop resilience. However, where the onset of the abuse or neglect of the child occurs from infancy and extends over time and is perpetrated by the child's carer or a family member, the impact of the trauma is complex and according to De Bellis and Zisk (2014) associated with greater rates of post-traumatic stress, depression and anxiety, antisocial behaviours, and greater risk for alcohol and substance use disorders in adolescence and adulthood. Their study indicates that the continued stress experience results in,

> elevated corticotrophin releasing factor (CRF) a key mediator of the stress response, causes generalized arousal, anxiety, aggression, hypervigiliance, and stimulation of the sympathetic nervous system (SNS), all core symptoms of the post-traumatic stress disorder (PTSD) hyperarousal cluster. It also causes inhibition of feeding and sexual behavior, core symptoms of major depression, another common outcome of traumatic experiences in childhood.
>
> (2014:5)

Of particular concern, according to Radford *et al.* (2011:87), is that,

> Children who experience abuse in childhood are more likely to be re-victimised by other perpetrators, including in adulthood, and those who experience multiple forms of abuse and re-victimisation tend to have the poorest outcomes.

Children and young people, whose early childhood lives have been defined by trauma, fear, and anxiety that they have never been able to communicate, find themselves being propelled by emotions of panic, rage, hopelessness, and helplessness. This can create what has been described as 'acting out' behaviour that is destructive and self-destructive. They find it difficult, sometimes impossible, to integrate good experiences in their life, and to learn from these, whilst being able to accept personal responsibility for their behaviour. So, how do we develop a way of helping children and young people to recover from their experiences of trauma, wherever these early experiences were situated, helping them to become more able to manage the external world of reality, without acting out or breaking down?

The book examines the following questions:

- After assessment and diagnosis, how can we move forward to treatment and intervention that addresses the emotional plight of traumatised children and young people?
- How do we help workers to engage emotionally when faced with the overwhelming behaviour of those for whom they are responsible? How can we enable them to become responsive, rather than over-reactive to the incidents they are presented with?
- What knowledge and understanding of therapeutic intervention do workers need if they are to engage with children and young people who have been labelled 'hard to reach' throughout their lives?

In addition to children, the term 'young people' is used to cover the age range 10–24 years as defined by The World Health Organization (WHO) and the United Nations (UN). Uniquely, the book explores different areas of work with children and young people in a range of contexts that comprise placements in residential care, fostering, adoption, young offender institutions, and council placements of unaccompanied minors seeking asylum. The legacy of early trauma is reflected in the impact on education, health, and life opportunities and forms part of the summary together with a discussion about potential ways forward.

The book is presented in two sections:

Section 1: From Theory to Therapeutic Treatment Plan introduces the fundamental building blocks that underpin the book, defining terms and examining the impact of trauma which is developed in Chapter 1 to examine attachment, fragmentation, and integration, and Chapter 2 which presents the heart of the book, the Needs Led Assessment and Therapeutic Treatment Plan.

Section 2: Reaching the Heart of the Matter extends the concepts and themes presented in Section 1 to show how they can work in a range of different contexts, which include residential care, secure provision, and unaccompanied asylumseeking children and young people. These are detailed and exemplified in the chapters that follow within the Needs Led Assessments, Therapeutic Treatment Plans and case studies that have been carried out by Christine Bradley, together with the guidance to workers and carers.

Chapter 1 focuses on attachment, fragmentation, and integration as an introduction to the chapters that follow. It examines how these concepts influence work with the children and young people in various stages of their development after considering the impact of traumatic experiences on their emotional development and on their future lives. This chapter will be presented in the context of three key stages of child development early years (0–6 years), latency (6–11 years), and adolescence (12–18 years) to lay the groundwork for the subsequent chapters and to examine how early traumatic experiences influence later maturational development. Infantile maltreatment can affect brain development, producing a brain that is focused on survival, at the expense of normal maturation and cognitive development. Traumatic and abusive experiences for the child during latency can result in their being more prone to risk-taking behaviours in adolescence, without the capacity to think about the consequences to themselves, or the negative outcomes of their anti-social behaviour. They are more likely to identify with criminal behaviour and substance misuse and with behaviour that is characterised by violence and conflict with parents, making their case histories more complex and distinct than those of younger children (Bowyer and Flood (2014); Taggart (2018)).

The cases presented examine how the legacy of maltreatment and trauma in children and young people's lives is expressed by them in their day-to-day living, and how the intervention of workers can impact on their behaviour.

Chapter 2 presents the Needs Led Assessment and Therapeutic Treatment Plan model, which is central to the chapters that follow and a unique contribution to the book. The chapter provides the formulation of the fundamental content of the inner working model of practice, giving workers a greater insight into the management of the child or young person discussed. The model comprises an assessment of the emotional needs of the child or young person followed by the creation of a personalised treatment programme which can support the journey of recovery from their earlier trauma.

The task of the Needs Led Assessment is not aimed at labelling the child or young person as having a specific mental health disorder but rather through carrying out a Needs Led Assessment, to offer a way forward. It enables workers to identify the fragmented aspects of the child or young person's emotional life with greater insight and understanding, specifically, the impact this has on their ability to manage reality and all that it entails. The assessment form within this chapter provides the basis for the formulation of the stage 2 treatment programme which is intended to identify the quality and nature of the support and provision needed, to enable the children and young people to deepen and strengthen their own sense of self.

The model for the Needs Led Assessment and Therapeutic Treatment Plan presented here, has been evolved and tested in practice over many years. It supports those who are working with and caring for deeply traumatised children and young people, helping them to feel emotionally stronger and more positive about their own sense of self, and to gradually work towards their future life with a sense of hope and belief. Assessing the emotional, cognitive, and social needs of these children and young people and identifying the extent of the fragmentation that exists in the child's internal world will help their workers and carers to respond effectively to the difficult and potentially destructive behaviour they present, and that prevents them functioning in the external world positively.

The Needs Led Assessment programme was first developed in the 1970s by Donald Winnicott and Barbara Docker-Drysdale in their pioneering work with adolescent boys transforming an approved school into a therapeutic community aimed at meeting the boys' emotional needs. The evolved model presented in this book has been developed and tested to meet the needs and demands of the 21st century and to provide workers with insight and understanding in handling the complexities of therapeutic work with children and young people. Examples of the assessment and Treatment Plans are presented within the chapter.

Chapter 3 examines how therapeutic treatment can make a difference to the lives of children and young people in residential care. The data show that just over 400,000 (3%) children and young people are in the social care system at any one time. The majority (74%) are of white ethnicity, 10% were of mixed ethnicity, and 8% were of Black or Black British ethnicity (Ofsted, 2019a). The task faced by carers in finding placements that address the needs presented by this wide range of children and young people who carry combined factors of ethnicity, and cultural and mental health difficulties is onerous. This chapter will discuss the key factors that are critical in creating a children's home which becomes a meaningful therapeutic environment, one that facilitates and can meet the emotional needs of traumatised children and young people.

There is an ever-increasing demand on carers and professionals to achieve a good outcome for children and young people who need specialist care and provision. The level of serious mental health issues in these young people is higher than in previous years, and consequently, the enormity of the professional task in the residential treatment of children and young people is difficult and extremely complex. If the work is to be valued and recognised as much as it deserves, it is important that workers and other professionals are helped to understand the difference between good childcare and therapeutic management. Central to this chapter is the capacity of workers to bear some of the most unbearable factors that emerge during the child and young person's day-to-day living. Without this critical insight and understanding, residential placements are in danger of delivering reactive and institutionalised practice, which does not reach out to meeting the emotional needs of those for whom they are responsible.

Chapter 4 explores how traumatised children and young people can be prepared for adoption, examining this from two perspectives, that of the adopted child and that of the adoptive parent. This chapter aims to help post-adoptive parents develop the insight and understanding to enable them to respond appropriately and with sensitivity to the young people they have adopted. Since many children and young people of adoptive families are overwhelmed by unbearable and unthinkable anxieties, their relationships with their new families are inevitably shaped by anxieties and fears which have resulted from the original trauma they experienced with their primary carer. The extent and impact of the trauma experienced can result in the child or young person being afraid to develop meaningful attachment relationships with the 'new' parent.

Adoptive parents play a critical role in the life of the children and young people and consequently require access to training and guidance to help them recognise what 'difficult to manage behaviour' means. Fundamentally, this is about understanding what it is that the child or young person is trying to, but unable, to communicate. Although the young person can present themselves as being 'fine' on the surface, the slightest stress can cause them to break down, especially where there is a constant fear or anticipation that their new family and adults will repeat their early experiences of trauma. To continue the transition to their new family placement requires guidance and patience. Without appropriate thought and support being given to both the child or young person and the parents, relationships can become increasingly stressful and escalate the acting out of increasing difficult behaviour that the parents are unable to deal with. Without timely and appropriate help and support, the adoption relationship can fall into danger of breaking down.

Chapter 5 examines the preparation of traumatised children and young people for long-term foster placement. Research shows the long-term vulnerability of children in care during their formative years identifying an increased mortality risk across ages 20–56 years (Gao *et al.*, 2017). Many children and young people in foster care are left with an inability to make significant relationships without behaviours emerging as a response to the unthinkable and unbearable experiences that they hold. This is often because their primary attachment left them overwhelmed with feelings of panic, rage, and a surge of anxieties which could not be thought about or expressed, and of being emotional abandoned rather than being held in the mind of their primary carer (Bradley with Kinchington, 2017). Consequently, as they start to attach themselves to their foster parents, the anxiety and panic which belong to their early trauma are in danger of being transferred onto and repeated with their new parents. This results in anxiety, insecurity, and ultimately unpredictability for them when forming a new relationship with a secondary parent. It is critical that foster carers have insight and understanding about what the child or young person's difficult behaviour represents, and how it can relate to the impact of their previous early trauma. The primary attachment figure in the child or young person's life can remain in their inner world of feelings and memories. Foster carers can experience negative projections and transference whose origins lie with this earlier figure, thrown onto them. Unless the foster carers have reached a level of insight and understanding about what the child or young person's difficult behaviour represents, it will be difficult for them to withstand it. Without the workers and carers being trained and supported to develop some insight about understanding the true causes of the child or young person's behaviour, the placement itself will be in danger of breaking down.

Chapter 6 examines the type of support needed to help unaccompanied asylumseeking children and young people to settle in this country. This chapter will look at the contribution of three specialist refugee charities whose primary task is to provide for and support the emotional, practical, and educational needs of unaccompanied refugee and asylum-seeking children and young people. These charities recognise that children on the move face many safety risks and concerns, from being separated from their families to the risk of sexual abuse and violence along dangerous travel routes. For unaccompanied children, the routes they take can leave them feeling particularly vulnerable to increased risks of becoming victims of child trafficking and sexual exploitation.

It will seek to provide insight and understanding from both perspectives, that of the workers and that of the young refugees themselves through a series of questions. How can workers engage with children and young people who have been severely traumatised because of the loss of family, identity, and country, and examine the complexities of successfully completing the essential therapeutic task required in their work? How do these young people manage to respond to workers who seek to support them when they arrive into a new country having experienced traumas including loss, violence, being attacked, and feeling that they are no longer being a part of the community they have grown up in? How do they manage the ambivalence that they feel whilst also managing their emotional fragmentation that the traumatic experiences they have endured during their journey have led them to?

Chapter 7 explores the quality of provision of young people who are placed in secure children's homes or young offenders' institutions. This chapter examines the incarceration of young people in youth offending institutions (YOIs) and the experience of young people placed in a secure unit under Section 25 of the 1989 Children's Act, and reflects on whether these are 'fit for purpose' and have the capacity to meet the therapeutic needs of these young people. Children and young people between the ages of 10 and 17 are subject to a family court secure order if they are at risk to themselves, to others or at risk of running away. The safety of the child is paramount. The intention of this chapter is to contribute to deepening workers' understanding of the underlying reason for delinquent and anti-social behaviour which results in children and young people being placed in a secure unit. The chapter examines whether a secure placement has the capacity to address the emotional needs of this group of young people helping them to acknowledge their own sense of personal responsibility, and to share the external world, learning from their experiences with others, without acting out through a delinquent merger. In contrast, children and young people who have broken the law and are sentenced will be placed in a young offenders' institution.

Frances Crook (2020) from the Howard League for Penal Reform reported that young people in young offenders' institutions are often deprived of human interaction with many kept in solitary confinement, with little oversight from workers and living in an inadequate regime with little human contact. It is little wonder, therefore, that these young people whose early traumas have left them with little or no sense of self which they value become overwhelmed with negative and destructive emotions. Without appropriate care and treatment, this can result in them self-harming and continuing to re-offend when they leave their secure placement. To address the complexity of needs, this chapter will examine the concepts of the 'frozen' and 'fragmented' children and young people, who cannot learn from their experiences and have developed their own sense of reality, which does not relate to the external reality experienced by others.

The task faced by those responsible in youth justice settings, young offenders' institutions, is both enormous and difficult. It is proposed that a key way forward is to enhance the knowledge and understanding of workers to enable them to engage therapeutically with the young people for whom they are responsible. It is only through the development of their own insight and understanding about the concept of integrated and fragmented states of mind in children and young people, that they are able to work constructively with this group of young people to achieve positive outcomes that are centred on meeting their emotional needs, and, in this way, to address recidivism.

Chapter 8 examines the role of schools in supporting the learning, education, and lives of children and young people, and offers detailed guidance to enable schools to contribute positively to meeting the needs of children and young people in the wider care system. It is the right of all children to have an education. School has a central role to play, but often children within the care system are invisible to the teachers because of their low numbers in school, poor dissemination of information, and often, that the children and young people themselves prefer not to be singled out, victimised or labelled as 'being in care' by their peers and teachers. The impact of a negative sense of self can result in their becoming resistant to learning, finding the school environment too difficult to manage, and often quite painful. They are unable to believe that they can learn from their teachers, are overwhelmed by the pressure in the classroom, especially where they have poor literacy and numeracy skills and a poor learner identity, and, inevitably, respond by becoming disruptive. Addressing this resistance to learning to provide appropriate support and encouragement, enabling the child to feel a sense of belonging, provides the starting point to learning and exploring their future potential.

Finally, the **Conclusion** brings together strands from each of the chapters and reflects on the legacy of early trauma on the young person's self-identity, health, and ultimately their life opportunities, and how this insight and knowledge can enable workers and carers to work with these young people with greater confidence and to work towards making a difference to their lives. It is intended that this book will provide a deeper understanding of the difficulties and complexities of life and living for children and young people whose lives have been overwhelmed by traumatic experiences of abandonment, hostility, and abuse from others. It will draw together key findings and recommendations and provides critical ways forward that support recovery, enabling this group of children and young people to feel more hopeful about moving on to the next stage of their lives, and to live with a stronger sense of self. This is what they truly deserve from us all.

It is hoped that the book will offer insight and help to those who are responsible for supporting the needs of emotionally frozen and fragmented children and young people who are weighed down by unresolved trauma, unable to 'reach the heart of the matter' and in danger of remaining isolated and emotionally broken throughout their lives. The task for those responsible for them is to help them to start to believe that they do matter and exist as a person in their own right, and to find a new starting point in their lives, to look to the future where the challenges of external reality become more positive and manageable.

Section 1

From theory to Therapeutic Treatment Plan

Chapter 1

Attachment, Integration, and Fragmentation

The chapter discusses how the breakdown of attachment relationships in an infant's early life prevents them from internalising positive infantile experiences that form the basis of their thinking and emotional life. Good early experiences provide a secure base from which the infant's own sense of self can begin to develop and grow. The biological function of the attachment bond between a parent and a child is to protect and to increase the chances of individual survival through the attainment of the proximity of a primary carer who is pre-occupied with meeting their emotional needs (Bowlby, 1973). Failure of attachment has far-reaching consequences for the child. The roots of this failure lie in emotional, physical, or sexual abuse and neglect by the primary carer so that the normal emotional, cognitive, and social development is disrupted, and the child put at risk.

Any traumatic experiences and maltreatment that young children are subjected to in their early years can interrupt and influence their maturational development if not worked through with insight and understanding with those who are responsible for them. To support this, the chapter will examine the specialist understanding needed by workers and carers if they are to help this group of children and young people to recover from their early traumas to the extent that they have the capacity for emotional and social independence.

This discussion will be framed by current theory and set within the context of three key phases of development comprising early years (0–6 years), latency (6–11 years), and adolescence (12–18 years).

Over the past 75 years, our understanding of the inner world of the child from infancy through to adulthood has deepened and we have come to realise that without the emotional pre-occupation and ongoing primary provision from their carer, children are vulnerable, and their sense of self is compromised. When they are subjected to maltreatment and traumatic experiences in their early life, their subsequent ability to adjust to the challenges and demands of the outside world becomes too difficult to comprehend and manage. To prevent such emotional damage, the role of parents and primary carers is critical at this early stage.

Parents who foster curiosity and exploration of the inner world of both self and others build resilience in a child's inner world which then enables them to thrive

DOI: 10.4324/9781003132882-3

in the outer world. So, relating to the world outside the self requires a parental
focus on the inner world of the child

(Cooper, 2018:39).

An infant that lives within a family setting that engenders a felt sense of safety
and emotional support has the potential to evolve a sense of self, learning what
is 'them' and what is 'not them'. This begins, according to Fonagy and Target
(2005:39), 'a journey of understanding their psychological self, the emergence of
which relies on much more than an infant's ability to organise their own experiences'. So, we must ask, what about the child whose experience is framed by
constant maltreatment and traumatic experiences in their infancy and early childhood? The child's response to the trauma experienced is one of fear and panic,
and they become overwhelmed by unthinkable and unbearable emotions and reactions towards themselves and those responsible for them. These emotions become
locked away inside their own internal world, unable to be communicated about
or worked through. They are left with feelings of vulnerability, and isolation with
little or no sense of 'self' with which they feel comfortable. Consequently, as
they grow older, their responses to experiences and elements in the outside world
(external reality) are hostile. These experiences and elements are interpreted as
destructive and attacking towards them, mirroring the early infantile relationship
with their primary carer.

The long-term prognosis for children and young people who have suffered early
traumas can be poor and emotionally debilitating. Not only has their relationship
with the outside world become fragmented, but also they are unable to regulate
their emotions. This results in their capacity to function collapsing, because their
'locked-away' emotions of panic, rage, and unthinkable anxiety emerge and engulf
them, thus preventing them from relating to the outside world. It is likely that without appropriate support and emotional containment from others, breakdown will
occur, and the dislike and fury within themselves will be 'acted out' and projected
onto others, often in a destructive or self-destructive manner. Further, adverse
childhood experiences have strong long-term associations with adolescent and
adult mental health risk behaviours, health status, diseases, and early death (Fellitti
et al., 1998:2019).

Workers and carers play a critical role by engaging in the slow process of helping traumatised and emotionally fragmented children and young people to move
towards achieving a sense of self and becoming a person, one with a true meaningful belief in themselves as an individual, with whom they feel more comfortable. It
is essential that workers are helped to develop a well-informed understanding that
underpins their ability to reach out, and respond appropriately, to the 'lost' part of
those for whom they are responsible.

Such a challenge for workers and carers brings up a key question: where is the
starting point from which workers and carers can begin the slow process of helping
and supporting traumatised children and young people to achieve a healthy sense
of being a person in their own right? Finding that inner person that young people

feel comfortable with, and from which they can begin to develop as an individual with a strengthening sense of self, is a primary task, and one which is very painful and at times difficult for workers and carers to achieve.

There is extensive evidence to show that a large proportion of young offenders and those with serious mental health problems have been exposed to a variety of traumatic experiences in their early life. Felitti writes that human development is powerfully influenced by emotionally traumatic early life experiences and that traumatic events of the earliest years of infancy and childhood are not lost but, like a child's footprints in wet cement, are often preserved lifelong. Time does not heal the wounds that occur in those earliest years; time conceals them. They are not lost, they are embodied (Felitti *et al.,* 2010:xiii).

Although originally the research into mental health difficulties was focused predominantly on emotional attributes relating to the mother-infant emotional pre-occupation, within the last 30 years, links between psychological and neuro-biological damage caused through childhood trauma have emerged, suggesting the development of maladaptive developmental behaviour in children and young people. It has been recognised that children who experienced prolonged exposure to severe trauma during sensitive developmental stages experience changes in cerebral development with negative mental health outcomes (Brewer-Smyth and Koeng, 2014). This makes it even more important that we achieve a much deeper understanding as to how we can begin to reach out and respond appropriately to the lost parts of these children and young people which prevent them from functioning in the outside world with a 'creative inquisitiveness'.

An important question for workers and carers, and one that will be explored within this chapter, is: how do we recognise in a young child when their behaviour and level of functioning do not correspond to their age and expected developmental stage? What do we understand by integration as compared to a child that is frag-mented? These points will be examined and then elaborated in the discussion of the three developmental stages each of which will be accompanied by vignettes drawn from practice.

The Integrated child

An integrated child is one whose early experiences gave them a strong sense of emotional containment and maternal pre-occupation from their primary carer.

> Attachment relationships in infancy fulfil an evolutionary role in ensuring that the brain structures that come to subserve social cognition are appropriately organised and prepared to equip the individual for the collaborative existence with other people for which his or her brain was designed
>
> (Fonagy and Target 2005:333).

Although their internal world feels enriched, they continue to require a great amount of support and care from their parental figure, and they are likely to still experience turbulent and stressful times and traumatic periods in their life. However, because they have developed cognitively, psychologically, and emotionally, they have the capacity to 'work through' their painful times and are able to learn from their experiences, to think about their emotions, and use them positively when socialising and relating to others.

Socialisation and mentalisation become a part of moving towards emotional integration, and consequently, an integrated child is more able to:

• Take part in group activities and join in with the team keeping to the rules.
• Regulate and communicate feelings of anxiety, uncertainty, anger, and stress.
• Learn from their very painful experiences.
• Begin to take on board the outside world with more certainty and confidence, as they develop.

Nevertheless, the infant who is beginning to integrate and develop emotionally, periodically still needs to re-experience absolute dependence on their primary carer as they start to experience a sense of independence.

The Fragmented child

In contrast, a child characterised as fragmented is one who did not experience a positive early attachment relationship with their primary carer, nor did they experience a parent who was consistently emotionally pre-occupied with them in their early years. This resulted in them feeling emotionally isolated, with little or no sense of 'self', so that their inner world of emotions is not linked in with their experiences of the external reality. Consequently, the boundary between fantasy and reality becomes fragmented and too confusing for them to manage. These children can become overwhelmed with feelings of panic, rage, and unthinkable anxiety. Central to this is that they did not experience the parent as allowing them to be 'absolutely dependent' on them and responding to their emotional needs, but rather reacted to them in a hostile manner. This frames their experience and expectations of external reality as being there to attack them, which can lead to them attacking back as a way of coping with the overwhelming anxiety and fear that they feel.

Under these circumstances although the child can function, they need a great deal of support, since they cannot hold onto experiences and the slightest stress in their lives creates breakdown in their day-to-day living. Their emotions are so raw and overwhelming that they cannot hold onto them because they have become cut off from their inner world of emotions. Aspects of reality become too unbearable for them, so they build up their own reality that they believe to be the truth. As a result, they find it difficult to learn from their experiences, and cannot think about the outcomes of their behaviour and their effect on others. They deal with it by believing that what happened yesterday no longer exists so that a repetitive cycle of difficult behaviour and the 'acting out' of it continues, until breakdown occurs. Without specialist therapeutic treatment, they cannot work through their raw emotions, and importantly cannot start to think about themselves. Their personal identity can easily fragment, and these fragmented parts of their personality and the accompanying emotional responses require specialist insight and support to begin the slow process of integration. This process enables the development of the child as a person, one who has the capacity to develop a view of the outside world with which they feel comfortable.

This chapter has shown how we can begin to recognise the depth of inner reality and its workings for the traumatised child, examining how unresolved and unrecognised painful early experiences which if not worked through, continue to burden, and overwhelm, impacting on lifelong development. Not only can this trauma have a detrimental impact on their maturational growth but can also result in serious mental health difficulties in later life. There is a need to recognise that the inner world of pain and fury from the child's early life leaves a far-reaching legacy into adulthood.

The early years: birth to five years

Extensive knowledge based on observation and research has emerged over the past 70 years about the impact of early trauma and stress on the early years of a child's development. The research and reflective work of Bowlby, Winnicott, and Piaget has highlighted a greater insight into understanding how we can identify and recognise the behaviour of infants and small children, showing that difficult and unresponsive behaviour can represent the failure of nurturing, unresponsive, and insensitive relationships with their primary carer.

Evolving research from neuroscience has shown that early experiences influence the developing brain of the infant. McCrory *et al.* (2017) report that an emerging body of work has indicated altered neurocognitive functioning following maltreatment. IMRI research had demonstrated that childhood maltreatment is associated with altered functioning in a range of neurocognitive systems including threat and reward processing, emotion regulation, and executive control.

Research on the biology of stress shows how major adversity, such as extreme poverty, abuse, or neglect, can weaken developing brain patterns in young children. A report by the Centre on the Developing Child (Harvard University 2016) has examined the impact of neglect in the early interaction between the infant and the primary carer on brain development, stating,

> This 'serve and return' behaviour continues like a game of tennis or passing a ball back and forth. If the adult's responses are unreliable, inappropriate, or simply absent, the architecture of the child's developing brain may disrupted, and later learning behaviour, and health may be impaired

(2016:4).

The work of earlier analytical thinking based on the observational studies of Winnicott, Bowlby, and others on the impact of early infantile trauma and anxiety, together with the findings from the Harvard Centre on the Developing Child, and the research of McCrory *et al.* on neuroscience, has shown that providing stable, responsive nurturing relationships in the earliest years of life can prevent or even reverse the damaging effects of early life stress with lifelong benefits for their learning, behaviour, relationships, and health.

There is an increasing concern about the high level of domestic violence, poverty, and emotional, physical, and substance abuse that young children are being subjected to, making the task of those caring for them difficult to manage. Recognition of trauma, understanding the behaviours that result from these experiences and having the knowledge and tools to work confidently with these young children, is critical. It is vital that we as workers and carers recognise the impact of early trauma and abuse in an infant's life, and critically, how the impact of this early trauma can be reflected in subsequent behaviours. The child's ability to relate and function with others in the nursery, classroom, and other care settings can only be supported through intervention, using appropriate tools of practice to help them to recover and prepare for the next stage in their life.

Being able to draw on the breadth of research available is essential in providing insight for the development of a deeper understanding and improved working practice, especially since the legacy of early childhood trauma may be manifested in mental health and physical disorders in adulthood. The team at the centre of Harvard observe that,

> What matters in early childhood can matter for a lifetime. To successfully manage our society's future, we must recognise problems and address them before they get worse, in early childhood

(2016:3)

The following description is an example of a young child who was showing signs of trauma and abuse in their nursery setting and how the practice of the workers was able to help the child work through their lack of belief in themselves.

Paul was referred to a family nursery when he was three years old after being excluded from a previous nursery placement because of his aggressive and disruptive behaviour. He was the middle child of three children in a household which was dysfunctional, and in which a high amount of domestic and physical abuse was directed towards the mother. Paul's behaviour had been modelled by his father, who had taught him to be abusive towards his mother by punching her. Consequently, although he was only three, Paul's mother was frightened of him.

When he arrived at the nursery door, he stood rigidly and would not enter through the door without warm responses and encouragement from the nursery workers. Once inside the nursery, he would spend most of the time on his own, neither being able to nor willing to play with his peers and share with them. When he did, he disrupted the group play and became aggressive towards them. Although he was aggressive towards his peers, he was able to respond positively and show some warmth to children who were younger than he was. An interpretation of this behaviour could be that it represented what he would like to have received from his parents in his younger years. Paul's emotions were so deeply buried inside him that he could not express himself, nor could he communicate about the anger and sadness that he was feeling. When stressed, instead of expressing himself through temper tantrums, as is expected of a three-year-old when learning about managing reality, he often had outbursts of panic and rage. An expression of panic and rage is different to temper tantrums, being a more primitive level of emotions relating to earlier infantile experiences.

With support, Paul was able to learn from the nurturing experiences and good management provided by the nursery workers, and after nine months, he was able to move on from the nursery. He became more able to manage boundaries with support from his workers when confronted with stressors which effected his functioning and behaviour.

I have found Paul to be an emotionally fragmented child, who, because of his early trauma, has been left with a sense of self that is emotionally raw and at times extremely fragile. He still finds it difficult to hold onto boundaries and learn from experience, and although he is now at primary school, he is unable to manage the classroom setting for long periods without breaking down so that he can only be contained there for a short period each day.

This example highlights why it is important that difficult behaviour in emotionally fragmented children is understood and responded to accordingly and that those caring for them have a long-term view of supporting their emotional, social, and cognitive development, which has remained dormant and emotionally stuck because of early privation and abuse.

The latency child: 6–11 years

The latency stage of a child's development starts around the age of 6–7 years and ends with the onset of puberty at 11–13 years. During this period, any early trauma that has lain dormant both psychologically and physically in a child's mind and body begins to emerge. It is crucial that the individual be allowed to resolve specific conflicts of living and being if they are to successfully transition to the next stage of their maturational development. During this time, the pursuit of social and academic activities which channels much of the child's energy into emotionally safe areas, can aid and support the child in 'forgetting' the highly stressful trauma they have previously experienced and help them to manage their current reality and is indicative of integration. This can prepare them to move towards the subsequent physical, sexual, emotional, and intellectual maturational stages of their development.

However, we must ask the question, what about the child who was exposed to unbearable traumas and conflicts in their early life prior to the period of latency that has never been dealt with? The impact of these early experiences can be that they have little or no sense of self-worth, or the capacity to explore the world and begin to understand about managing reality positively. Consequently, they expect failure and negative experiences to shape their lives. When workers respond to the child's behaviour with confusion and frustration, the child, attuned to these emotions, picks up the feelings and, because they are unable to separate the past from the present, starts to experience the worker or carer as the same person who was destructive, hostile, and abusive towards them in their early years. This can result in the child attacking back either destructively or self-destructively, as their capacity to manage the realities of the outside world becomes too difficult to manage, reaching a point at which they can break down. Their life becomes a pattern of anti-social behaviour, mental health disorders, manic-depressive anxieties, and other diagnostic categories, which shape the reality of their life.

The following is an example of how a child in the latency period can start to recover from the trauma of his early experiences.

Jack is ten years of age, the eldest of four children, one brother and two sisters. The family were described as chaotic, and non-functioning, and where the children experienced a high amount of physical and emotional abuse with no safe and secure containment available either physical or emotional. Eventually, all the children were placed together into foster care. Within a few months, the placement broke down for Jack, mainly because of his drive to control his siblings, at times aggressively. This was because as the oldest child in the family, and since the level of parental control was being almost non-existent, Jack felt the need to become the parent figure to his siblings. This meant that he became the 'caretaker' for the family, leaving no space for him to be the 'lost child' that he experienced as a nine-year-old. The little self in Jack came to a standstill whilst he became the parent figure. Putting himself to one side prevented him from developing his own emotional strength and confidence and interrupting his physical and emotional maturational development.

Jack was placed in a children's home to which I was their therapeutic consultant. The Home had developed ways of assessing the emotional needs of children and young people they were responsible for and had gained a growing reputation for delivering individualised Treatment Plans to aid their emotional recovery. After Jack's assessment programme had been completed, it became clear that the extent of the trauma, deprivation, and abuse Jack had been exposed to in his early years had left him overwhelmed by emotions of panic, rage, and unthinkable anxiety and led partly, to his drive to control his siblings. Further, the assessment and treatment programme provided an insight and understanding about the roots of his aggressive behaviour. Despite the devotion and commitment that he felt towards his siblings, during their shared early traumas, Jack felt that as the oldest child in the family, he had to become the parent figure (caretaker/parentified) in the family. However, because Jack had also experienced significant early trauma, the results were that in his day-to-day living experiences he functioned partly as an older child in charge of his sisters, whilst at times he acted out his experience of life as the emotionally lost child he felt as an infant.

He still held onto emotions of panic and rage in his own inner world which at times resulted in Jack becoming quite aggressive and violent. I suggested that because the team recognise that because he felt that his mother had not been able to think positively about him, and constantly became over-reactive to him because of her own mental health difficulties, it was crucial he experienced his key workers in the team as constantly holding him in their mind. Allowing Jack to play and interact as he should have done as a small child, rather than needing to become a parent figure to his siblings, would enable him to hand over the lost 'little self' he carried inside him to his carers, permitting them to become his 'caretaker'. This could result in Jack allowing the little boy inside him to reach out to the team for the appropriate provision to meet his needs.

In my discussion with the team, I put forward to them that what Jack needed, if he were to allow them to break through to the little boy trapped inside him, was to ensure that he was able to experience a sense of emotional containment and safety from them which was not provided for by his family. To enable the appropriate therapeutic provision he required to help him to strengthen emotionally, they focused on providing him with appropriate play opportunities, together with the provision of good primary experiences on which he could allow himself to draw on.

The patience, stability, and insight the Home provided were central to reaching the trapped part of Jack and resulted in his own sense of self-strengthening. The team developed their own insight and understanding about meeting his needs and were able to provide appropriate opportunities for Jack, helping him to work through his past traumas. He was provided with a climbing frame outside the house together with a den, which he could take himself to when life in the children's home became too stressful for him. They also provided him with a kitchen and a doll's pram, together with a set of six teddy bears that he carried everywhere. These activities gave him the opportunity to play out his experience at the family home when he had to look after his siblings.

As Jack began to break through the mechanisms that he had put in place to help him survive, he became more able to work through and play out his experiences which occurred whilst he was living in his complex home situation. Also, he began to become dependent on his workers who provided for the lost child in his inner world, by reading stories to him, always running his bath, and becoming nurturing to him when preparing him for his bedtime.

After some months of focused play opportunities, and primary provision, Jack began to explore his fears and anxieties about his education, sexuality, and friendships. He is now beginning to understand more about his past trauma and the influence it has had on his maturational development. The real self in Jack has begun to emerge and strengthen in a more positive way than when he first was placed in the home. Whilst there is still more work to do with him, he is now in a position where his real self is now positioned in the latency period, rather than being trapped and locked away in a small child.

This case study provides an example of how it is possible to help severely traumatised children and young offenders to recover from their experiences in a therapeutic environment which can understand and facilitate their emotional needs. However, this can only be achieved where the team of workers have the insight and understanding as to how to meet specific needs which arise from missed early experiences. It is also crucial that to help the child work through some of their unbearable fears and anxieties, their level of communication with each other is positive and supportive. Importantly, the team themselves need to have the appropriate support, supervision, and consultation to help them work through what it means to live alongside severely traumatised children and young people. The development of Jack has shown the impact of this process on the team's skills and insight and self-reflection.

Adolescence

Adolescence is viewed as the transition phase from middle childhood into adulthood and evolving independence with the capacity to manage the pressures and challenges of life. It is a period during which emotional, physical, sexual, and cognitive development takes place, where personality and personal identity mature, and adult bonding relationships occur.

Winnicott (1965:87) makes an important point about adolescent transition, noting that this is a period when, to feel real, young people must survive the depression which he refers to as 'struggling through the doldrums'. An adolescent who is emotionally integrated will inevitably go through difficult periods in their transition from child to adult, at times 'struggling through the doldrums' but will have the resilience and capacity to work through these periods and come through to the other side. In contrast, the fragmented child because of the pain and anxiety they have been holding onto because of emotional and physical trauma experienced in their early life will lack the resilience and capacity to navigate this period of change. Adolescents whose early life experiences manifest themselves in difficult and reactive behaviour, which they cannot manage or understand, find the transition into adulthood difficult. They may struggle with anxiety, depression, low self-esteem, and, because of a fragmented educational experience, poor educational expectations.

Adolescents who leave care are particularly vulnerable and at greater risk of experiencing mental health conditions. 'Become', the charity for children in care and care leavers, recorded that in 2019, 12,560 young people left care in England aged 16, 17, and 18, with a further 26,990 leaving the care system aged between 19 and 21 years. Khan (2016) stated that approximately 10,000 16–18-year-olds left foster or residential care in England, and of these,

> 62% of care leavers were originally taken into care because of neglect or abuse, that only half of children in care had emotional health and behaviour that was considered normal; care leavers were five times more likely to self-harm in adult years (National Audit Office, 2015); 25% of those who are homeless have been in care at some point in their lives; 22% of female care leavers became teenage parents and 49% of young men under the age of 21 who had come into contact with the criminal justice system, had a care experience
>
> (2016:12)

To gain a deeper understanding, the differences in the behaviour of integrated and fragmented adolescents will be examined and compared in relation to two key aspects, namely, relationships with adults and groups, and managing emotions and reality. This will be followed with case studies of two fragmented adolescents (Table 1.1).

i Relationships with adults and groups
ii Managing emotions and reality

The examples below of fragmented adolescents in care show the importance of how being understood and responded to, with meaning and sincerity, by those responsible for them is central to their growth towards adulthood. Being listened to

Table 1.1 Relationships between adults and groups: contrast between integrated and fragmented adolescents

Integrated Adolescent	Fragmented Adolescent
Most adolescents who are emotionally integrated have been through some experiences of trauma during their life whether separation, loss, or a feeling of failure. However, because they have internalised a sense of good early experiences, they can battle through the pain and anxiety they hold and think about their future. Although they find themselves depressed at times, they are able with help and support to work through it all and find a way forward in their life. As they have been working at separating from their primary relationship, they are exploring themselves as an individual with their own sense of self, forming meaningful relationships with their own group of friends with the ability to take part in group activities and function within them.	In contrast, the fragmented adolescent finds meaningful relationships difficult to find and hold onto. Since their early experiences of absolute dependence on their primary carer did not occur, they constantly try to build relationships which are as intense as those they were denied in their early primary relationships. This can make it difficult for the other person to respond accordingly. It also leaves them vulnerable and subject to being seduced, to identifying with the anti-social tendency, gang crimes, and sub-culture with others. Their early trauma can easily be repeated, and this leaves them exposed to risk-taking behaviours and exploitation because of their need to seek out a sense of love and security from others.
Although they will disagree and argue with others, they will be able to work through these, returning to their relationships, carrying personal responsibility for their actions, and learning from their experiences.	
As their relationships with others develop and grow, they will begin to cover a wide range of peers. Within this part of their adolescent lives, they will start to form more intimate relationships with others, which involves not only sex but also holding, caring for, and sharing trustworthy relationships with others, and being supportive when facing difficult factors in their lives.	

and understood has been shown to enable the young person to develop a stronger sense of self, and importantly to internalise their workers' responses, as a good and positive experience. This experience is central in enabling the young person to manage and work through difficult and painful periods in their life, and leaving them, critically, with a sense of hope about their future (Table 1.2).

Table 1.2 Managing emotions and reality: contrast between integrated and fragmented adolescents

Integrated Adolescent	Fragmented Adolescent
An integrated adolescent has achieved a sense of self, and of being an individual. If they are emotionally integrated with enough sense of self that they feel comfortable with, they can find their place in society. Although they will have powerful emotions of anger, sadness, and loss, they will be more aware of how they are feeling and be able to express themselves, and work through these emotions. This in turn makes them emotionally stronger and able to face the challenges of reality they must manage. They will test the boundaries they have to face whilst being able to learn from their experiences.	Most fragmented adolescents were not able to express themselves in their infantile years. Often, the reactions from parent figures were ones of hostility and attack rather than being emotionally containing and holding. This can lead to emotions of panic, rage, and anxiety, which they cannot think about, and can result in them being unable to relate to the outside world with a sense of interest and aliveness. Their sense of emotional isolation and early abandonment makes it impossible for them to manage the challenges of the reality faced in their life. They 'disconnect' from the outside world, as they cannot bring together their emotions, which are embedded in their inner world to connect positively with external reality. Consequently, the outer world becomes unbearable and unthinkable for them to manage. Although they seek to find a way of surviving external reality, the emotional vulnerability they are holding can take the form of more perverted, primitive, and challenging behaviour, which can lead the adolescent to over-identify with the cultures of the anti-social tendency and even re-creating their own reality to follow. These behaviours can have a long-term impact on their life choices and chances.

Ben was placed in a therapeutic community for boys when he was an adolescent. He came from a family situation of multi-generational deprivation and emotional privation and inadequacy, which is the case for most young people who require special looked-after provision. He had appeared before the children's court several times. Although his placement at the therapeutic community was mainly a positive one where he felt that he received genuine and meaningful provision and responses from his workers, it did not end positively, and he drifted into a difficult and anti-social period in his later years.

Critically, he clearly internalised enough good experiences from his placement in the Home that he was able to contact one of his ex-workers several years later. He felt it important to inform him that their support of him was vindicated and recognised. Although he did go through some difficult times in his life, he had received enough good experiences during his placement at the Home and that he was now very settled with a family and ongoing work.

Ben's experience shows a journey interrupted through trauma, but one that he was able to continue himself because of the impact of the early intervention that he received from his placement. He showed that he had the capacity and resilience to continue his journey to recovery, managing to overcome difficulties and adapt, even where at one point he was involved in risk-taking behaviours. He had the capacity to reflect on his experience and, in the early days, to regulate emotions of anger and panic by self-medicating. The relationship and intervention he received from his key worker had an impact that he carried with him, rising to the challenges of adulthood with success through a long marriage, a successful family, and continuous employment.

Ann was a 16-year-old adolescent who had experienced a difficult morning, but I was delighted to enjoy the opportunity of spending some time with her. She looked serious and thoughtful, and knowing that she had experienced a difficult morning, I asked her how she was feeling now. She told me that she had thought about killing herself and jumping in front of a train but did not have the courage to try. She then said that nobody believed that she tried to jump in front of a train. I pointed out to her that it did not matter whether she did or did not; what really mattered was that she was in such despair about herself that she could not see a way forward and wanted to end it all. That is where the workers at the Home could help her. The following are the key points which emerged in my talking with Anne and were central to where she was at that moment in time in her life.

She has been beaten up in the past, and the memory was very much alive in her mind and easily re-enacted, and even though she was not physically beaten up, metaphorically she explained that she felt beaten up in school the previous week.

She was desperate to feel listened to and felt that she was not always taken seriously by her workers. I explained to her that that her carers took her very seriously and were deeply committed to helping her. Perhaps it was because she sometimes found living with herself quite unbearable, which made it difficult for them to be able to respond to her appropriately all the time.

I reassured her that they were most prepared to learn more about how they could begin to understand her emotions when she presented herself like that.

When unhappiness and despair came over Ann, she felt very lost, and her emotions became extreme and dominated her thoughts. These emotions resulted in her wanting to hurt herself or others, emotionally and sometimes physically.

She was very aware that at times her actions could be serious, but because she did not know how to deal with her emotions, she cried, and although she could not feel anything without becoming overwhelmed, when she cried it was a way of expressing herself to others, but even then, it did not always feel real. I replied that because she had been able to express herself to me, it suggested that she was a very real person, who was trying to find her own way through surviving really difficult times, although with great difficulty. I assured her that the staff team in the Home were more than committed to supporting and helping her to become strong enough to manage the difficult and painful times she sometimes encountered.

Finally, Ann told me that she was really worried and frightened about having to leave the Home in two years' time. She was afraid of having to face the outside world on her own, and two years was not enough time for her to become strong enough to believe that she could manage it. I replied that in this situation, it was most important that the staff team and she made the best use of the time they have with her to help her to manage herself, in the best possible way.

I found meeting Ann and having the discussion with her a truly inspirational and moving experience. Although in many ways her placement at the Home has been a successful one, she still is exceptionally emotionally raw and at times very fragile. The therapeutic relationship of the team with Ann must focus and respond to her on two levels, namely, as a 16-year-old who is having to accept the reality of the outside world and learn how to manage living there, and the other part of her that is still functioning like a five-year-old, who is anxious and afraid of the outside world and sharing the world with others.

The emotional containment Ann has received from the Home has helped her to develop and strengthen some aspects of her day-to-day living. However, if workers do not help her to begin to feel better about herself in other aspects of her life, she could be in danger of breaking down when she leaves the Home. The areas that need to be addressed are: (a) the parts of her day-to-day living when she finds functioning difficult and painful, and to help her to continue functioning; and (b) for workers to acquire a deeper understanding, as to the roots from which her non-functioning emerges. This insight needs to be followed up with the therapeutic provision and support she requires if she is to develop and grow with meaning and with an inner strength from which she will be able to manage the outside world.

The short case studies presented in this chapter help to illustrate the complexity of these young lives and indicate the extent of the long-term work required by experienced workers with a psychotherapeutic understanding when they are supporting the emotional, social, and cognitive development of these young people towards adulthood. The chapter has attempted to portray the pain, hurt, and lack of holding onto a secure sense of self-esteem that traumatised children and young people are forced to carry with them throughout their lives, if not provided with the appropriate therapeutic responses from those taking care of them. It is crucial that we build up enough insight and understanding from their workers to enable them to recover from their experiences. The next chapter will focus on the development of a pathway towards ongoing recovery.

Chapter 2

Assessing the needs of traumatised children and young people and creating a Therapeutic Treatment Plan

Introduction

The previous chapter has examined the differences and similarities between children and young people who have been through traumatic experiences in their early years in contrast to those who have experienced emotionally secure early bonding and attachment relationship with their primary carers. With appropriate support, children and young people can work through the fears and anxieties that they have internalised because of traumas experienced. The impact of trauma on a child or young person who did not develop a meaningful and secure attachment relationship with their primary carer and was subjected to reactions of emotional abandonment, hostility, constant abuse, and trauma, is overwhelming. This experience results in the child feeling emotionally fragmented, unable to bring together the different aspects of how they feel about themselves and leaving them unable to integrate further experiences. They expect the trauma of their earlier years to be repeated, a pattern characterised by anticipated ongoing hostility and aggression from others. Without appropriate help and therapeutic treatment, they can view the outside world (reality) as being there to attack them, which they respond to, by attacking back. The long-term outcome for them can be poor and sometimes negative. Trowell and Miles (2011:34) reported that,

> The incidence of depression in children has increased markedly over the last few years. Children do not just get better of their own accord. They go on to lead limited lives, under achieving at school, at risk of consuming drugs and alcohol and finding themselves increasingly in social isolation, suffering repeated depressive episodes. If these children have symptoms of anxiety, their prognosis is all the more worrying.

This chapter aims to enable teams of workers who are directly involved with traumatised children and young people, to provide individualised care and treatment through the use of the emotional Needs Led Assessment and a planned treatment programme. The process is designed to enable workers to address and understand the symptomatic behaviour of those for whom they are responsible, and critically,

DOI: 10.4324/9781003132882-4

to deepen their understanding psychologically so that they can understand, relate, and respond to the child or young person's inner world of trapped emotions which exert a controlling influence on their day-to-day life. The assessment programme designed for the individual child or young person will help identify the specific aspects of their emotional development which prevents them from functioning positively, because their early trauma has left them emotionally fixed at an infantile and early childhood stage of their maturational development. The process of carrying out a Needs Led Assessment and Therapeutic Treatment Plan enables workers to reach out to the unbearable feelings of hopelessness and helplessness that the child or young person carries within them and respond appropriately. The task is to work towards reaching a positive outcome for the traumatised child or young person, enabling them to find a point at which they become more able to manage the challenges of external reality without breaking down, and move towards becoming more integrated as a person with a stronger sense of self and psychological development than that initially displayed.

Since 2015, the current Needs Led Assessment programme and Therapeutic Treatment Plan model presented in this chapter have evolved to define a route through which enables workers and carers to help children and young people whose trauma remains emotionally trapped, and not worked through by them. The effect is that their sense of self is 'emotionally fragmented' with many aspects of their personality being 'split off' into their unconscious leaving them unable to balance out internal and external thoughts and feelings about themselves and to function as an integrated person. Consequently, they are unable to cope with life and make healthy relationships with others, and because they remain emotionally vulnerable, they are more susceptible to anti-social behaviour and delinquent tendencies. Their behaviour is characterised by a failure to conform to social norms, a lack of remorse, and little sense of being able to accept personal responsibility for their actions.

The original version of the Needs Led Assessment programme and Therapeutic Treatment Plan was developed in the 1970s through the pioneering therapeutic work of Barbara Dockar-Drysdale, Dr Donald Winnicott, and Richard Balbernie with emotionally damaged children and young people and brought together and tested out in the work of the Cotswold Community in Wiltshire. Although originally an approved school for young people, it eventually transformed into a successful therapeutic community working with young offenders who had often failed in other placements. The impact of their innovative practice with the use of Needs Assessment and Treatment Plan programmes was that after ten years they were able to show that recidivism (young people returning to young offenders' units or prison) dropped from a previous 85% when it was a formal approved school, to 0.5% after it changed becoming a therapeutic community focused on meeting the emotional needs of the children and young people for whom they were responsible.

The importance of the Needs Assessment and Therapeutic Treatment Plan programmes has been recognised, and, since its original format some 50 years ago, has been adapted to fit in with the current needs and demands of work with traumatised children and young people. Importantly, the underlying philosophical underpinning of the work has not been lost and continues to provide the 'heart of the matter' and the basis for insight and understanding by practitioners who provide therapeutic treatment for work with emotionally fragmented children and young people.

Definition of terms of assessment

The terms used to characterise the assessment of trauma of children/young people are presented in a sequence, which ranges from pre-attachment with the frozen child or young person moving towards the fragmented child (archipelago) and the parentified (caretaker) child or young person, through to fragile integration and on to ego-integration with the development of positive attachment relationships, characterised by a stronger sense of self, purpose, and individuality.

The Frozen child

Everyone experiences traumatic events; however, it is not the occurrence of the trauma but how the individual deals with a traumatic event, which determines the impact that it will have on their lives (Vaccaro and Lavick, 2008). If left unresolved, the feelings surrounding the trauma can persist, impairing judgement and effectively freezing the child or young person into harmful patterns of behaviour, including sexual risk-taking, and being unable to accept personal responsibility for their behaviour.

For a child who was not able to progress beyond their earliest experiences of maternal care, they remain fixed in a state of seeking 'maternal unity' with their primary carer. They are unable to separate and view the external world with interest because they are overwhelmed by the traumatic experiences of abuse, hostility, and emotional abandonment faced in their early days. The result for the frozen child is that they constantly seek to recreate the primary merger with others. This makes it too difficult and painful for the child to make a healthy attachment relationship, because they have not yet reached the critical stage of pre-attachment and the point where they can begin to relate to people. They can become overwhelmed with feelings that they cannot bear to think about or understand; consequently, emotions of panic and rage begin to emerge, leading them to behave in a destructive or self-destructive manner towards others.

Critically, the child or young person learns how to adapt to others without it having any meaning to them. The maltreatment and trauma experienced in their early years can result in repetitive states of behaviour constantly being displayed in their day-to-day living as they cannot manage the stresses and challenges of external reality. It is all too easy for their daily lived experiences to become a repetition of their original trauma, creating a situation where they 'act out' their unbearable emotions and which inevitably results in the disruption of reality and relationships in their lives.

A frozen child can present a superficial charm, which leads workers to think that they are in a solid functioning emotional state. The dissonance is that at times they can be extremely friendly and make good contacts very quickly, but a minor upset, or disappointment, can result in them flying into panic and rages for no apparent reason, becoming savagely hostile, smashing, and destroying anything in their vicinity. The volatility of their emotions is at such a primitive level in their unconscious, that a minor misunderstanding in their daily lives can return them back to their early trauma, which remains unresolved and 'frozen' in their mind.

Guidance for workers

The frozen child cannot manage boundaries and finds group experiences difficult because of their need to merge with an individual, so the child can only function as part of a group if they have an adult with them. When they do attach to their workers, they recreate their need for a primary merger, when two people become one. Having not yet reached a stage of two people attaching, once they do attach, they merge *(enmeshed attachment)* to become a part of that other person. Workers need to be aware that as a frozen child begins to depend on them, they need to ensure that the child knows that they are being held in mind, understanding that separation is too difficult for the child to manage.

If good primary experiences are provided for them continually, they can develop a strong sense of absolute dependence on their worker and the continuity of the relationship and their sense of self will strengthen them sufficiently to the point where they will be able to engage in group experiences and adhere to agreed rules.

The child or young person who cannot manage their emotions and has low self-esteem and will needs constant encouragement from their workers. If they have been positive in their actions, let them know how much their actions and achievements are valued. It is important for the worker to recognise how difficult it is for the child to value themselves. If they can be aware that you recognise their painful feelings, it will help them to continue to function, and to realise that you are prepared to take care of them until they can look after themselves.

A survival mechanism is not a way of helping the child or young person to cope with anxiety. It is mainly a reaction to unbearable and unthinkable feelings. A healthy defence mechanism helps to reduce anxiety in the child as they are protecting their sense of self.

It is essential for the worker to recognise whether the child has left them feeling anxious or worried about them. At this point, it is important to let them know that you have been thinking about them since you last met. The fact that you were left feeling concerned about them suggests that it is likely that they are feeling horrible about themselves. Respond by asking whether there is any way you could help them prior to them feeling that they can no longer control themselves.

Create as many opportunities as possible for the child to communicate at a non-verbal and symbolic level. Using too many words could make them feel attacked. Remember acting out can be a breakdown of communication, which needs to be understood and addressed symbolically.

The child or young person needs one-to-one help. It is important to be aware of their emotional rawness and fear of breakdown, which could occur, and to communicate this to them. Support them by helping their challenges of learning through small, simple, and manageable stages. They need to be aware that you are prepared to learn with them. The child needs opportunities for sensory play. Whatever their age, they could benefit from receiving some good primary play experiences including playing with puppets; storytelling; and reading books or writing stories with each other or with a person who they feel emotionally contained by and who can survive their need to annihilate their play (McMahon, 1992:10). They need to have a reliable time each day when they play with a specific adult, who they can depend on, using their play opportunities in ways which can help their emotional development.

Fragmented (Archipelago)

The term 'the fragmented child' (described in the work of Donald Winnicott as an 'archipelago' child) is characterised by a legacy of abuse, neglect, and trauma, and although appearing superficially as integrated, the child may manifest signs of being internally fragmented. The impact of this early trauma and the consequent disruption caused to their maturational development results in the child trapped in a fragmented world of areas of functioning and non-functioning (Bradley with Kinchington, 2017). The concept of an archipelago fits well with the explanation given by Dockar-Drysdale (1990) who described traumatised children as 'being made up of ego-islets that never fused into a continent'. What she meant by that was that because of the overwhelming anxiety that their traumatic experiences filled them with, they were unable to develop a secure sense of self which could allow them to manage the challenges of reality encountered in their lives.

Although the child has the capacity to function positively for short periods, this is not a stable situation. They hold onto a deep-rooted sense of self-loathing and alienation, and, consequently, view the outside world as being there to attack them. Critically, when their level of functioning ceases, they can develop a 'false self' that is effective in pretending to others that they are functioning well. Fragmented or archipelago children and young people are deeply emotionally fragile. It is the worker's and carer's primary task to develop ways of responding to them which helps them to eventually believe and feel themselves to be a person and an individual, able to function creatively, and begin to make sense of and understand the outside world. As they begin to develop the capacity to ask for emotional support and containment when they start to feel vulnerable, they will start the process of functioning, and strengthening their sense of self in their day-to-day living without having to use the 'false self' to pretend to others that 'all is well with them'. Undoubtedly, a fragmented or archipelago child is filled with 'internal struggles' which, without appropriate provision and response towards them from those responsible for their care, are in danger of falling into a continuation of emotional fragmentation, with large missing gaps of functioning in their day-to-day living.

These gaps characterised by the internal struggles and the child or young person's behaviour could lead to a misdiagnosis of conditions such as bi-polar disorder or psychosis. It is crucial that workers and carers can identify and assess their level of functioning which can easily break down and recognise the precursor danger signs which accompany breakdown. They must also develop the necessary insight and understanding needed if they are to provide appropriate therapeutic treatment programmes to aid the child or young person's emotional recovery from their trauma and help them to think more positively about themselves. The aim is to help the child or young person to move towards reaching a level of ego-integration with their own sense of self becoming emotionally stronger, and more able to share the world with others positively and constructively.

Guidance to workers

Workers must be careful not to idealise them when they are functioning and expect this to continue indefinitely. When the child or young person's functioning does break down, it is important not to express disappointment to them; respond but do not react. When their functioning diminishes, this could be the time when they require structured primary provision from their carer. Workers need to help the child to realise that they recognise how difficult and painful they are finding it to manage their current difficulties. Provide them with an experience at a primary level, which will help them to feel looked after rather than emotionally abandoned.

Workers need to remain in touch with the child when they begin to show a deep sense of anxiety, which is becoming unbearable. At this stage, it is important not to react to them as this will feed into their fear of being attacked by the outside world, leading them to act out. Let them know that you are aware they are worrying about themselves. Suggest that perhaps you should both find a quiet space where you can sit down with a drink and biscuit to talk about what is making them feel so terrible. Then, you can think about a way in which you can help them to feel better. Ensuring that they know that their worker is in touch with some of their own unbearable feelings will make them feel a little more hopeful about their current difficulties.

Provide as many opportunities as possible for them to communicate symbolically; use stories or painting to provide them with creative ways to communicate. If workers can stay with the child's despair and self-destructiveness, they protect them from their more primitive impulses and so emotions feel less raw. As their sense of self begins to develop again, they will be more able to communicate through words about how they feel. The child or young person needs one-to-one help. Workers and teachers need to be aware of the pain and despair they can reach if they continue to repeat past experiences. Identify the length of time they can be expected to function in a challenging situation. Ensure that your expectation of what they can achieve is presented to them in small stages, building up to a point where they are ready to undertake more challenges. They need opportunities for transitional play using a cloth, a toy, or a blanket, which provides the child with a sense of protection from the outside world. With the use of a transitional object, the child can move forward to the use of symbolism in their play stories, drawing and music. It is through these types of play experiences that the archipelago child may be able to communicate and relate to their fears and anxieties, and importantly, the use of a 'transitional object supports the child engaged in the perpetual human task of keeping inner and outer reality separate yet interrelated' (Winnicott, 1971:2).

The Parentified child (Caretaker)

Parentified is a term used to describe invisible childhood trauma where a child has had to grow up too soon because of the failure of positive parenting by their primary carers. It is apparent where a parent-child role reversal takes place requiring the child to take on a caretaker, mediator, or protector of the family role. Children who have been robbed of secure early childhood experiences and placed in a situation where they have had to invent themselves as adults in charge of the other children find themselves with a gap in their psyche. They harbour unbearable early emotions of anger, grief, and a sense of emotional abandonment within themselves which can unexpectedly at times 'burst' out. The parentified child is unable to think about how they are feeling, because their own emotions are too overwhelming for them. They have been so busy caring for siblings, or the emotional needs of parents who are unable to see the needs of their child, that they have lost their own sense of self, and the capacity to function as an individual in their day-to-day living.

Winnicott (1958) described the importance for a child to experience significantly good experiences in their early years, from a carer whether a mother, father, a foster carer, grandmother, an aunt, or a period in a specialised residential setting. This ensured that they had formed an attachment relationship with a primary carer internalising some good experiences. However, where the child then experienced a separation at this point, before they were ready to let go of their identification with their carer, the sense of loss is profound. The loss of their carer traumatised them to the extent that they were unable to attach to another individual unless they were in a position of looking after them, instead of being able to take care of themselves. This traumatic experience of loss impeded their developmental growth and resulted in the child having to become their own 'caretaker'. Although emotionally fragile when managing the challenges of reality and the outside world, the child can be reached emotionally by others through communication either verbally or symbolically. Even though the child can be prone to wild temper tantrums and a deep sense of sadness and loss, nevertheless, they can still be supported and protected from acting out feelings of panic and rage.

To assess the emotional needs of the parentified child and provide for them accordingly, it is important that workers and carers can recognise the 'little self', who is trapped inside the inner world of the child or young person and allow the handing over of the 'caretaker self' by the child to the worker or carer. This would enable the lost child to be provided for and cared for by their worker and accept a feeling of being cared for themselves. This would help the 'little self' to feel looked after again, and to psychologically develop and mature as their own sense of self starts to feel more contained and nurtured. The experience could help them to strengthen their sense of self-esteem, to become more aware of their strengths and weaknesses, and to begin to value themselves. The positive outcome of sound therapeutic treatment is that the parentified/caretaker child or young person is given the opportunity to developmentally reach the point of 'emotional integration'. This enables the child to share the world with others and make a place for themselves that they value and enjoy.

Guidance to workers

Let the child or young person know that although you do understand why they must be so controlling, it would be more helpful if they allowed you to take care of them, as you are aware that they are very anxious and worried. The worker becomes the caretaker, leaving the child to be the little self who needs looking after.

A parentified/caretaker child is more able to accept personal responsibility for their actions than other children who are deeply unintegrated. When their workers notice that the pressure is building up inside them, they need to let the child know that they are aware that they are becoming anxious and unsure about themselves. Suggest that that the child or young person finds a quiet space where both can sit and talk about how they are feeling.

The worker needs to help the child to hand the caretaker over to them to be looked after, and to provide for the little self who needs to be taken care of. At this point, the provision of good experience being adapted to meet their primary needs for a short period of the day becomes important, for example, a cuddly object they can communicate with, a drink, or special food with their workers. There is a part of their self, which continues to feel emotionally contained by their workers, until they acknowledge that they no longer require the provision.

Offer as many creative opportunities as possible for them to symbolically communicate such as drama, story writing, poetry, painting, and music. This allows the symbols to become the third object of communication, making it easier to eventually find words to express themselves. The child or young person requires a one-to-one situation to help them to want to learn. There is the potential to learn, but they need a great of emotional support and help to believe that their carer (in the form of an adult or teacher) recognises the vulnerability of the 'little self' and has the ability to respond to their fears and anxieties, helping them to feel taken care of and, in doing so, increase their desire to learn. Ensure that they have several play opportunities at both an infantile and chronological level as their play offers opportunities for them to communicate and to be creative.

Fragile Integration

A fragile integrated child has a greater awareness about the importance of boundaries than unintegrated children. Under stress, they are more likely to challenge and become anti-authority as they are beginning to accept personal responsibility for their actions and become part of a group. Their ability to manage boundaries influences the group dynamic. Either they can help the group to function or under their own stressful periods, can disrupt and prevent it from functioning. Although the sense of self in the fragile integrated child is stronger, they can manage stress factors only for a short period. Their emotional resources are not yet strong enough to hold onto their self-esteem continually. Fragile integrated children can communicate symbolically. They are reaching the stage of emotional development where they can begin to express themselves verbally but require some help with their communication. At this stage, they will be ready to use therapy. Workers need to remain aware of the level of their communication and the point at which they cease to communicate.

Fragile integrated children are either committed to learning or resistant to being taught. This depends on the dynamics of the classroom influencing the sense of security the child has within the setting. Fragile integrated children are in a stage of transition from being without a sense of personal responsibility with a lack of guilt and concern, to focusing more on a sense of doing and learning and making reparation for their destructive behaviour. Stress can result in them returning to their points of breakdown when they were unintegrated. A child who is working towards a level of ego-development and a strengthening sense of self is now able to think about the stress they are under and needs opportunities to communicate with their workers about their difficulties. Workers need to respond sensitively towards them, helping them to reflect on what the learning experience means. As they begin to realise what they can gain from their learning environment, it will help them to take in the experience and link in more positively with the reality they are working with.

A child at the stage of fragile integration is more able to play with others and keep to the rules, although at times, they need more symbolic and creative play. Play can be used as a greater form of imagination with them, projecting and working through some of their more painful feelings and memories through it. Children at the stage of ego-integration begin to differentiate between fantasy and reality. They can use their play environment to work through some of the difficulties they experience when balancing the realities of their external and internal worlds, which can become instinctually rich or poor. Winnicott (1971:44) observed 'Integrated children have moved and directed from the state of not being able to play, into a state of being able to play'.

Guidance for workers

The following four areas are central to therapeutic work with fragile integrated children and young people:

Personal responsibility: As the child or young person moves towards integration, their sense of self begins to strengthen and they build up a greater awareness about their actions. The attachment relationship between the worker and child develops, enabling them to acquire a sense of reliability and trustworthiness for their actions. As they begin to come together as a person, with help and support they can begin to show greater accountability for their behaviour and slowly to gain control for their actions. The worker must then focus on the child's personal identity and sense of self, helping them to achieve a greater sense of personal responsibility.

Disintegration: Even where the child or young person begins to come together as a person, they are not yet emotionally strong enough to manage difficult and painful experiences in their day-to-day living. If the pressure of the outside world feels too much for them, they begin to view the outside world as a dangerous and threatening place to be in and start to feel attacked by it. At this point, they retreat to their inner world and are in danger of disintegrating and returning to their point of breakdown. Workers should respond sensitively and thoughtfully to them, helping them not to give up on their ego-developmental process. Acknowledging that an episode of disintegration will lead to a coming together could make them feel stronger.

Communication: Offer as many opportunities as possible for the child or young person to communicate particularly about the stress of managing reality. Support them to invest in their level of communication when they are trying to face their challenges. Follow the level of their communication; if it diminishes, the acting out of difficult behaviour is likely to occur. Always remain in touch with their quality of communication. Express your concerns when you view their positive behaviour as being in danger of breaking down and ask them if you can help them in any way. At the level of fragile integration, the child still needs to know that they are held in mind.

Transference and countertransference: As the child or young person begins to feel a person with their own sense of self, they start to transfer some of their emotions, which arise from experiences and traumas with previous figures in their lives, onto their workers. To work positively with the transference dynamic, workers need to acquire some insight and a deeper understanding of this key concept.

Carrying out a Needs Led Assessment and creating a Treatment Plan

The Needs Led Assessment and Therapeutic Treatment Plan are presented as a **four-stage model** (Figure 2.1) and comprise sets of key questions related to different syndromes of disorganised attachment, comprising frozen, archipelago, or caretaker, and present the starting point for the team in working therapeutically with the child or young person.

The Needs Led Assessment and Therapeutic Treatment Plans are designed to understand and address the symptomatic behaviour of an unintegrated child or young person. This process helps to identify the level of privation, deprivation, and trauma, which has been experienced in the child's early life and examines how these experiences have influenced and prevented the young person's emotional and cognitive maturation.

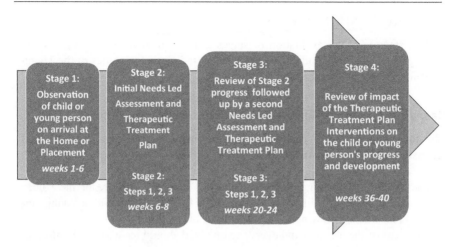

Figure 2.1 Relationship between the initial observation of the child or young person and the Need Assessment and Therapeutic Treatment Plans.

The assessment framework followed by a Therapeutic Treatment Plan identifies the quality of support and provision they require if they are to recover from their traumatic and abusive early experiences. This offers the team a starting point and indicative diagnosis, which enables them to ascertain whether the child or young person has reached a given point, and, critically, the direction they need to travel in if they are to recover from their point of breakdown. The scope of the intervention and contingency plans must be thought through so that the young person is supported throughout should a breakdown occur. Carrying out the Needs Led Assessment and Therapeutic Treatment Plan also helps the team to identify the knowledge, understanding, and skills they require, to support the child or young person to progress beyond the point of breakdown.

Stage 1: OBSERVATION

Stage 1 comprises a period of the child or young person on their arrival at the residential Home or foster placement.

Stage 2: THREE-STEP PROCESS

This three-step process involves carrying out an initial Needs Led Assessment, asking key questions to identify the potential initial indicative syndrome, and developing an appropriate Therapeutic Treatment Plan. These three steps form an integrated package, the results of which can then be used to inform stage 3.

Stage 3: REVIEW OF STAGE 2 AND MODIFICATION OF THERAPEUTIC TREATMENT PLAN

Stage 3 draws on the outcomes of stage 2 to inform the process of carrying out stage 3, which follows the same three-step process as stage 2.

Stage 4: EVALUATION OF IMPACT

This stage uses the evaluation of stages 2 and 3 to review the progress and development of the child or young person based on the outcomes of the Therapeutic Treatment Plans carried out earlier.

Carrying out stage 2: initial Needs Assessment

The following guidance is advised in carrying out the stage 2 Needs Led Assessment, which follows the observation period.

- The assessment meeting should involve all workers who are or have been engaged in the child's life over the six weeks following the child or young person's placement following the initial stage 1 observation.
- The chair of the meeting and everyone involved should have as much information as possible about the first few years of the child's life, their relationship with their primary carer, and any significant events.

The Needs Led Assessment should only be carried out when the child or young person has been in their placement for six to eight weeks to ensure that as much information has been gathered about the child or young person in terms of their background and them in situ in the placement.

- Not all the questions on the assessment form (Table 2.1) need to be asked, but rather the most appropriate three or four questions should be identified, to help the meeting (lasting approximately two hours), to acquire a deeper understanding of the needs of the child.
- The meeting often views the child as fitting into different aspects of the syndromes of deprivation. It is normal that there should be a variety of thoughts and ideas from professionals in the meeting. The syndrome that brings out the strongest agreement in the meeting about the child should be the one to be used as the focus for the Therapeutic Treatment Plan.

Step 1: Key questions that help identify an appropriate assessment

The team of workers are asked to consider and respond to the questions listed below in relation to the individual child or young person that is the focus of the Needs Led Assessment. There are seven categories, which need to be considered, accompanied by sets of key questions that are central to the Needs Led Assessment. The categories comprise in general: boundaries, merging and functioning; containing, emotion, anxiety, anger, and stress; self-destruction and self-preservation; communication; and learning from experience and play. An affirmative response to the questions relates to an indicative characteristic of one of the three potential assessments of frozen, archipelago, or caretaker as classifications of fragmented/disorganised attachment.

Table 2.1 Identifying the potential indicative assessment: the relationship between categories, questions, and indicative assessment

Phase 1 Category	Question	i. Answer Yes or No. ii. If Yes – Give an Example or Explanation for this Decision	If Yes – Initial Indicative Assessment
1. Boundaries, merging, and functioning	1. Does the child merge and disrupt the functioning of others?		**Frozen**
	2. Does the child have any areas of functioning?		**Fragmented/ archipelago**
	3. Is help needed when functioning breaks down or can the child manage stress and transitions?		**Fragmented/ archipelago**
	4. When under stress does the child merge and disrupt the functioning of others?		**Parentified/ caretaker**
2. Containing, emotion, anxiety, anger, and stress	5. Can they contain emotions, or do they act out violently?		**Frozen**
	6. Do they act out violently when under stress?		**Fragmented/ archipelago**
	7. Do they react violently under pressure or perceived threat?		**Parentified/ caretaker**
3. Self-destruction and self-preservation	8. Do they have very low self-esteem and cannot take care of themselves?		**Frozen**
	9. Under stress can they take care of themselves, or do they show a range of symptoms from self-mutilation to suicidal gestures?		**Fragmented/ archipelago**
	10. Can they protect themselves? Is their self-preservation haphazard?		**Parentified/ caretaker**
4. Communication	11. Can the child talk meaningfully in a one-to-one situation, or do they just chatter without meaning?		**Frozen**
	12. Is there the potential for some communication, but they back off when anxious or stressed?		**Fragmented/ archipelago**
	13. Does the child communicate in a way that is not easily understood and often symbolic?		**caretaker**

(Continued)

Table 2.1 (Continued)

Phase 1 Category	Question	i. Answer Yes or No. ii. If Yes – Give an Example or Explanation for this Decision	If Yes – Initial Indicative Assessment
5. Education, and learning, from experience	14. Can the child learn from their personal, social, and school experiences, including mistakes?		**Frozen**
	15. Does the child have the potential to learn, cognitively and emotionally through communication, but lose it under stress?		**Fragmented/ archipelago**
	16. Does the child find learning at school a difficult experience?		**Parentified/ caretaker**
6. Play	17. Has the child ever learnt how to play?		**Frozen**
	18. Is the child's play easily distracted and sometimes destructive?		**Fragmented/ archipelago**
	19. Can the child play, but at an infantile level?		**Parentified/ caretaker**
7. Fragile integration	20. Can the child hold onto boundaries, but push them in an anti-authority way, especially under stress?		**Indicative assessment: fragile integration**
	21. Do they disintegrate when very anxious and are unable to talk about stress?		
	22. Under stress do they lack self-esteem and self-care, can they become self-destructive?		
	23. Is communication more at a symbolic level with little investment in verbal communication?		
	24. Do they find it difficult to face reality and when out of communication, break down into anti-social behaviour?		
	25. Does the child have a general commitment to school, and the experiences which are offered to them?		
	26. Does the child engage in solitary or cooperative play?		

Step 2: Interpreting the potential initial indicative assessment

Total the number of responses in the right-hand column of Table 2.1 and summarise in Table 2.2 below:

i It is likely that a range of indicative assessments will be identified; however, the highest number of responses within a single box will give you an indication of the most relevant assessment of the child or young person.

Step 3: Developing an appropriate Treatment Plan

i Prioritise three areas from the list below that the team feel need to be worked through as a matter of priority with the child or young person. These will form the focus of the child or young person's Therapeutic Treatment Plan set out in Table 2.4.
ii Completing the 24-hour care Therapeutic Treatment Plan

Transfer the three priority areas from Table 2.3 onto the template below (Table 2.4). Read through the responses and exemplars that you have listed initially in Table 2.1, and use the 'Definition of Terms of Assessment guidance to workers' in the section 'Definition of terms of assessment', to help the team to interpret the assessment and to create an appropriate Treatment Plan based on the priorities identified for the child or young person.

Table 2.2 Summary of responses to identify indicative assessment

Fragmented/ archipelago	Frozen	Parentified/ caretaker	Fragile Integration: Yes/No

Table 2.3 Identifying priorities to create an appropriate treatment plan

Treatment Plan Category	Indicate Priority
Boundaries, merging and functioning	
Communication	
Containing emotion, anxiety, anger, and stress	
Learning from experience and education	
Play	
Self-esteem and self-preservation	
Fragile integration	

Table 2.4 Creating the 24-hour care Therapeutic Treatment Plan

Category	Therapeutic Treatment and 24-Hour Care Plan

Stage 2: Creating the follow-up Needs Led Assessment and Therapeutic Treatment Plan

A follow-up Needs Led Assessment meeting on the individual child or young person should take place during weeks 20–24. The three-step process is repeated as for stage 1 and focused on building on the progress made during stage 1.

This re-focused 24-hour Treatment Plan is aimed at supporting the continued development of the child or young person within a given time period.

Stage 3: Evaluation of the Therapeutic Treatment Plan intervention

The evaluation that takes place during weeks 36–40 is critical. It enables the team responsible for the child or young person to review the impact of the Therapeutic Treatment Plan interventions on the child or young person's progress and development, from the beginning commencing with the initial observations and Needs Led Assessment, through to this point in time. It allows for professional discussions about the young person's progress and development and to plan for future actions and potential intervention.

Section 2 of the book: Reaching the Heart of the Matter and the case studies in the chapters that follow illustrate how the use of a Needs Led Assessment and Therapeutic Treatment Plan programme is able to offer the insight and understanding that will enable workers to provide a therapeutic focus to their work with the children and young people that will support their emotional and maturational development.

Reaching the Heart of the Matter

Chapter 3

Making a difference

Therapeutic treatment and practice
with young people in residential care

Introduction

This chapter examines how a sense of self can develop and mature in children
and young people placed in specialist therapeutic residential care settings. This
difficult and complex task shows how a meaningful therapeutic environment
impacts on young people and the workers responsible for them. It exemplifies
how the work carried out can meet the emotional needs of traumatised adolescents and how it can contribute to the slow process of addressing the impact of
early trauma. The case study is based on the Needs Led Assessment and Therapeutic Treatment Plan presented in Chapter 2. The recommendations are followed
with my reflective account following a one-day placement in the young person's
Home which has an embedded therapeutic culture. Carrying this out has provided
a deeper insight into both the internal and external life of the young person, and
the support needed by workers who live alongside and work therapeutically with
him. The focused specialist training and consultation that have taken place over
the years in the Home have given the workers the confidence and understanding
about working therapeutically with children and young people who are placed
with them.

   As part of the wider context for the case study, it is important to review the
range of care settings in England and to examine the impact of being in care on
both the traumatised young person's emotional development and long-term survival and, critically, the stress experienced by workers living alongside these young
people. Inadequately trained or inexperienced residential care workers are unable
to provide therapeutic care that addresses the complex needs of traumatised young
people whilst maintaining their own health and professional confidence. The cost
is not only to the young person, but also to care workers' burnout resulting in their
leaving the profession, and ultimately to society where unresolved mental health
issues force young adults back into health and care systems and the juvenile justice
system.

   Ofsted reported that as of 31 March 2020, there were 2,378 children's Homes
in England, with over three quarters run by private companies (1,815); 408 by

DOI: 10.4324/9781003132882-6

local authorities; and a combined 155 by trusts, voluntary providers, and health authorities providing 10,033 placements for children and young people (Ofsted, 2020:11). Residential care can be viewed as a spectrum that ranges from Homes that offer childcare where basic needs of shelter, safety, stability, food, and care are met, to ones that, exceptionally, provide this within a therapeutic environment. Although many residential Homes may claim to offer a therapeutic environment, the ones whose philosophy and practice are centred on therapeutic care are few and far between. Understanding the difference between good childcare and therapeutic management is critical, since without the insight and understanding that this brings, residential placements default to delivering institutionalised care that is reactive in response and that is unable to reach out to meet the emotional needs of the young people for whom they are responsible.

The impact of developing nurturing relationships for the young person is profound. Wijedasa et al. (2022:5) reported that

> Children and young people in care who had positive relationships with their carer(s), friend(s) and social worker(s) were more likely to have better mental health, irrespective of the length of time they had spent in care or the number of previous placements they have had. This highlights the importance of ensuring the continuity, stability, and quality of relationships with key people throughout children and young people's time in care.

The effect on workers living alongside children and young people whose lives have been defined by trauma cannot be underestimated. Research suggests the impact of vicarious trauma on those working with survivors of traumatic life events (Bloom, 2003). Psychological boundaries and the way that the residential Home cares for its workers are critical if workers are to manage stress and resist burnout which leads to high staff turnover. The Australian Centre for Excellence in Therapeutic Care (CETC, 2019) in their intensive therapeutic care manual for managers and supervisors states that,

> The development of secondary traumatic stress is recognised as a common occupational hazard for those working with and caring for traumatised young people. In therapeutic residential care, there is a close connection between the young people and the staff. This relationship exposes the worker to the distress and pain experienced by these young people, yet it is strengthened through empathy and a strong desire to alleviate the pain and suffering. Residential houses invariably include young people who are living with the impact of trauma, loss, violence, fear, poverty, depression, hopelessness and helplessness and a wide range of other physical and mental health issues
>
> (CETC, 2019:35).

The reflections of living alongside a young person such as that presented here offer insight and guidance for the training and development of the staff from the perspective of an experienced practitioner. It provides a deeper understanding into the depth of insight and knowledge that residential workers require if they are to work therapeutically with children and young people. Their task is complex, and they require appropriate support to ensure that they are successful in producing a good outcome for the young people for whom they are responsible.

It is inevitable that workers in children's Homes are likely to come across complex cases of children whose background is characterised by trauma, loss, and arrested emotional development. To support workers, two key elements have been singled out that will enable them to maintain their professional boundaries and to bear the stress of the powerful emotions generated by their work without their burning out. These areas of knowledge relate to transference and countertransference and that of being a reflective practitioner.

i Transference and Countertransference

Transference is the process whereby a child displaces onto the worker feelings and ideas which derive from previous figures in child's life; countertransference is when the workers take on the behaviours to 'become' that person. If not thought about and worked with, it can result in the child experiencing the workers as though they were the original attacking person, and this can create more destructive or self-destructive acting out of their emotions through their behaviour. It is important that workers are given the opportunity to reflect on how they are left feeling after having spent time with specific children, critically to recognise how much of the emotions they experience have been projected onto them, and how much is what being with the child has brought up emotionally for the worker themselves. An understanding of projection is critical since without understanding and insight, the worker is vulnerable to projecting their own unexpressed and unbearable feelings onto the child in response to what the child has projected onto them.

ii Developing reflective practice

At the end of each day, the staff team should come together to discuss how they are feeling having been with specific children all day. Articulating their own positive or negative emotions will give them an understanding of the emotional life of the child and provide an opportunity to reflect on the impact of intensive therapeutic work on a day-to-day basis. Diamond (2017) has highlighted the importance for workers to have the space and the opportunity to reflect on the impact of such close work with young people.

It is important to recognise that it can be painful and difficult for workers to manage working with specific children whose inner world of reality is so emotionally fragile. Importantly, the Needs Led Assessment and Therapeutic Treatment Plan guidance offers a starting point that will enable the team to develop their understanding and therapeutic practice through such a complex case.

Case study: Harry

Background

Harry is a 13-year-old boy who had been exposed to continual trauma of emotional and physical abuse, hostility, abandonment, and rejection throughout his early years. His chaotic experiences had been exacerbated by inappropriate and inadequate therapeutic and physical care within a series of establishments ranging from unregulated children's Homes to secure and young offender units. The lack of emotional containment in many of the placements has resulted in his behaviour spiralling out of control and his becoming destructive towards others and self-destructive towards himself. As a result, Harry was sectioned under the Mental Health Act (1983) in a psychiatric hospital, and eventually placed in the children's Home where I met him.

As a result of the extent of the traumatic experiences that he experienced, Harry has not been able to internalise a secure space in his own internal world of emotions and thinking. He is a deeply 'fragmented' child, whose sense of self is extremely fragile. To survive, Harry has built up a 'false self', developing a persona for himself to protect against re-living traumas that he experienced in his earlier life. The false self is a façade for living which does not allow for authentic spontaneity and fun in his day-to-day life. Closely observed, his behaviour is controlled and engagement superficial, even though he may present as charming and social to the onlooker. The extent of the emotional pain within him has left his inner world unfeeling and empty. Under pressure, his body language becomes stiff, and he is unable to speak without twitching and blinking his eyes, behaviour that becomes more pronounced as he tries to control himself and repress his overwhelming emotions of panic, rage, and despair.

Harry has built up some strong 'dependency relationships' during his stay at the Home, particularly so with his key worker with whom he has become absolutely dependent, rather like a small child. However, his behaviour fluctuates so that at times he presents himself like a 13-year-old boy, and at others as a lost three-year-old still seeking his missing early primary experiences and unexpressed emotions trapped inside him.

Harry: Needs Led Assessment outcome

Following the Needs Led Assessment, it was agreed to focus on two dimensions that were central to Harry's Therapeutic Treatment Plan and critical to supporting integration and ego-functioning, and the development of Harry's self-identity:

1 Containing emotions of anxiety, anger, and stress.
2 Self-esteem and self-preservation.

1 Containing emotion, anxiety, anger, and stress.

Harry lives in a constant state of anxiety of trying to please people. His previous experiences were of adults reacting to him in a hostile manner, and his fear was that if he did not meet other people's expectations, the traumas that he has experienced in the past would be repeated. He has shown for the first time at the Home that he has the capacity to become 'absolutely dependent' on workers who reach out, provide, and meet his needs. However, he is not yet ready to make a secure attachment with them, because the 'lost child' in him still needs to have his primary needs provided for and met.

Harry presents as a fragmented (archipelago) child, with aspects of him which can function, but which are so fragile that the slightest stress factor can lead to repeated breakdown in his day-to-day living. This leads to his depression and despair emerging, preventing him from functioning. He holds small areas of functioning, which must be valued by his workers. However, he can easily fall into areas of chaos since he expects failure and attack and so requires a great deal of emotional containment to help him survive his unbearable sense of loss and fears of abandonment.

2 Self-esteem and self-preservation

In this category, Harry was assessed as functioning at the level of a 'frozen child'. This relates to the earliest parts of the infant's existence and where his experiences were full of emotional abandonment, with a lack of holding, containment, and ongoing nurturing by his primary carer. Consequently, the centre of his inner world became 'frozen' so that he was only able to function at a superficial level, becoming increasingly susceptible to breaking down and acting out his unbearable emotions (Bradley with Kinchington, 2017). Harry had no belief in himself as a person in his own right because his emotional life remained frozen and buried inside him. Importantly, as there was no basis from which he could develop a secure attachment with others, he experienced the outside world as being hostile and painful to manage. To survive, he created his own reality about what was going to happen to him. Harry's inner reality is based on an empty shell defined by trauma and feelings of hopelessness, helplessness, and worthlessness. He places no value on himself, and consequently, he is unable to take care of himself.

The small child in him needs to be able to live through the sense of absolute dependence on people he can trust, at which point he can then start to take care of, and value himself and, importantly, find a new starting point for his own developmental growth. His education has been as inconsistent and unreliable as have his placements, and so consequently, he finds learning quite a frightening experience and expects the worst to happen to him.

Therapeutic Treatment Plan

Harry is an extremely complex young person who has not yet found his own starting point in terms of his emotional developmental growth. The team's support is key in facilitating his development. He has not yet approached the phase where he could make meaningful attachments with his workers. However, it is important to note that the team have made him feel more emotionally contained than any of his previous placements.

It is important to recognise that because Harry's early experiences were ones of such extreme privation, his responses are very primitive and that when he begins to live alongside workers on whom he is dependent, they will find it personally quite emotionally painful as they gradually come in touch with the depth of his despair. It is important to realise that it is only through meaningful therapeutic work that in time, Harry can begin to feel more real and reach a point where his own sense of self can start to grow. The aim of therapeutic work with Harry is to help him reach a point of 'fragile integration' within the next 12 months, and for him to become more able to move towards managing meaningful attachment relationships with members of the team.

The following points are critical:

1   Being held in mind

Being 'held in mind' describes the emotional attunement and empathy towards the infant by the mother (primary maternal preoccupation) which enables the infant's transition into the autonomy of being a separate person (Winnicott, 1960).

For a child who has been as deprived and traumatised as Harry was in his infantile years, it is crucial that he experiences 'being held in the mind' of those caring for him as he is still at a very early stage of his emotional development. To enable this fundamental experience to occur, workers need to be able to consistently respond to Harry with a deep understanding as to how difficult and painful life can be for him at times. This will help him to feel that the environment is being emotionally nurturing to him, which could help him to develop a more positive outlook on life, and to begin to restructure his relationship with life and living. Harry needs to have short, but complete experiences with a worker on whom he is dependent. Discussing the areas that made him very anxious and not wanting to learn are important as this could help him to feel that he really does matter to people who continue thinking about him.

2   Support his day-to-day living

Harry's capacity to function throughout the day under stressful situations is at risk of disintegrating and falling apart, preventing him from functioning. This can lead him to becoming overwhelmed with feelings of hopelessness and helplessness. It is important that workers do not have too high expectations of him in his day-to-day living. The part of Harry which is a teenager needs to be supported in functioning whilst the aspect of his self who still feels like a small lost child needs providing for, in a structured way. Think of what he needs you to provide for him at important parts of his day: in the morning to help him face both the day and his school day, because he finds transitions difficult to manage, and finally in the evening to help him talk about his night-time anxieties.

3   Managing his emotional fragility

Harry is a deeply emotionally fragile young person, and because he does not have the emotional resources to help him deal with managing the internal stress factors in his day-to-day living, it is too difficult for him to communicate about the daily hardships he experiences. When he feels let down or emotionally abandoned by situations, he can react angrily or attack others. Where a stressful situation can result in him feeling very insecure, it is important that his workers help him to take personal responsibility for the situation. This will enable him to learn how to manage the stress until he is able to accept personal responsibility for himself. Let him know that you are aware when he is feeling anxious and worried about a situation by asking whether there is anything that he needs from you to help him. It is important that he has the opportunity to communicate about how he is feeling at the present time.

4 Communication

Communication is a key factor in therapeutic work with Harry. However, it must be recognised that he will not yet be ready to communicate verbally about his anxieties. He requires as many opportunities as possible for other non-verbal ways of communicating including symbolic communication through play and art. It is anticipated that he may be ready to use child psychotherapy shortly.

A personal experience of working with Harry

The day I spent with Harry took place when the team was two weeks into using the Needs Led Assessment and Therapeutic Treatment Plan programme created for him. I had met him once before and briefly explained that I would like to come and spend a day with him in the Home, would he mind that? He was most excited that somebody would like to spend time with him. When I arrived at the agreed date, he opened the door to me. Although he was pleasant and controlled, I was aware that he was showing extreme anxiety and a sense of uncertainty towards me. He became quite fidgety and then walked away to the other side of the house. He was unable to communicate with me until I had been there for some time before he was calm enough to sit down to speak with me. Harry had been on his own with another boy of his age during that week as the younger children in the Home were on a week's summer holiday with some of the working team and due to return later that day. I asked him how he was feeling about life in the Home without the younger children present, and he replied that he enjoyed being there only with the other boy present because he received more continual attention from his workers when the younger children were not there. It was clear that although Harry wanted attention from adults, he was also afraid of feeling annihilated by them, because these emotions are what he often experienced during his earlier life.

What I experienced in the day I was with Harry was that although he acknowledged my presence and responded to me, it was difficult to truly engage with him and to communicate in any meaningful way. I concluded that although he feels emotionally contained and positively responded to and accepted in the Home, which is crucial for a starting point with him, he is unable to let go of the powerful emotional impact of his earlier traumas. His own sense of self is so complex, and he has become emotionally raw over the years that although he has become very dependent on his key worker, his need for attention and recognition remains at a very infantile and early years' level. It will take some time for Harry to be able to make an attachment relationship in which he feels secure, either with her or other workers, one that carries a true meaning for him that he will begin to internalise and develop emotionally. It is only at this point that he can start to transition from being dependent on them and move towards becoming more inter-dependent and begin to feel like an individual in his own right with his own sense of personal identity. It is important that workers reflect on not allowing Harry to build up a 'false self' during therapeutic work with him.

I explained to Harry that I would be leaving at an earlier time than originally planned, because the young children were arriving Home later that afternoon, and it would have caused disruption for somebody they did not know being there. He came to see me out and help me move my car from the drive. I said that I had thoroughly enjoyed spending the day in his Home and thanked him for being so friendly. I felt very emotionally moved by Harry and the other child in the Home. It was also another great realisation for me as to what a complex task the therapeutic treatment of children and young people in residential care who have been deeply traumatised can be, and how difficult and painful it can be for the workers at times.

There are four areas of practice to be thought about in the therapeutic treatment of Harry:

i Reflective practice

The need for reflective practice by residential workers is crucial to enable them to develop the awareness, skills, and understanding to manage some of the unbearable emotions working with seriously traumatised children can bring up for them. Having the opportunity to discuss their feelings and responses with other workers can offer opportunities to share practice and responses to children's behaviour and importantly to strengthen their boundaries and resistance to projection and countertransference.

ii True and false self

The false self can be used as a defence against emotions that are unthinkable. If the true self feels exploited, the individual will feel annihilated and locked away from functioning, which could lead to serious breakdown (Winnicott, 1960). The environment that Harry grew up in did not facilitate normal emotional maturation. The real self in Harry is overwhelmed by anxiety and uncertainty and which if not worked with in a therapeutic environment, and responded to appropriately, could result in emotions of panic and rage not being able to be thought about, but instead be acted out, either destructively towards others, or self-destructively to himself in the future. Dockar-Drysdale (1990:47) observed that the false self in children emerged because their experience of primary deprivation resulted in their evolving 'a tiny real self' which was contained in 'a shell of adapting to demands, which others make on them'.

iii Managing transitions

Harry needs to experience relationships which enable him to become 'absolutely dependent' on his special workers, which he is currently beginning to show. He then needs his workers to use their own insight and understanding to help him to manage the transition from this absolute dependence to a stage of being inter-dependent with them. This will only occur when he has developed a sense of self which is strong enough, and where he has enough belief in himself to manage the outside world of reality successfully.

iv Communication

It is important that Harry can begin to express himself verbally which will enable him to start to think about his emotions. In his early days at the Home, Harry found it too painful to express himself verbally because he was not yet able to think about his emotions. To deal with this, he began to build up a false self, remaining in denial about the hurt and pain he had experienced and about his fears and anxieties which he held onto when having to manage the reality of his day-to-day living. It is not only psychotherapy that will help to meet his emotional needs, but also the culture and philosophy of the Home that will reinforce his daily experience and help him to communicate, and, importantly, help him to recognise that he is being understood.

Outcome of the Needs Led Assessment and Therapeutic Treatment Plan programme

My meeting with Harry's key worker took place six weeks after the Needs Led Assessment and Therapeutic Treatment Plan programme was put into practice in the Home. The aim was to review the outcome of their use of the assessment and treatment programme on the emotional growth and development of Harry's maturation during the time it was being put into practice.

It was felt that Harry's sense of self, which is full of anxiety and uncertainty, is now developing and becoming more real and he is more able to express to others how uncertain he is about his future, even though he maintains that he is still not yet ready to talk about his feelings. This is a positive step forward. Further, he is about to have a trial day with the local air cadets' organisation which he would very much like to become a part. If he is accepted by them, it will be the start of Harry making a transition from his need to be dependent on the team at the Home, and to begin to strengthen his own sense of self becoming more able to manage reality factors in his life more positively.

However, more inexperienced members of the team find their experience of working with Harry painful at times and difficult to manage. Although he can be charming to be with, they are also aware that he carries a high amount of more primitive emotions in his inner world, which consist of panic and rage and which, without appropriate responses, can result in his behaviour becoming more destructive or self-destructive to himself and others.

It was agreed that Harry's true real sense of self is beginning to emerge rather than staying within the 'false self'. He is now more able to express some of his more painful feelings for a short period, when with a worker on whom he is dependent. His key worker has been working on providing an experience of provision for him which is aimed at meeting his primary needs. For example, when he returns Home from his school day, she provides him with a cup of tea and a biscuit, and they find a quiet space where they can discuss the day which helps him to express some of his worries and concerns about how his day has been.

The other aspect of the therapeutic treatment of Harry over the past 6 weeks was the emergence of Harry's transference relationship with workers. He is quite desperate to have a family to which he feels that he belongs. Currently, he sees the Home as a family, and some of the workers as parent figures, with his key worker, in particular, as a mother figure. The team acknowledge the importance of recognising Harry's need to feel that he is a part of a family. Whilst his key worker understands that being recognised and taken seriously is crucial and important to Harry, she also recognises the importance of holding onto her own professional boundaries in Harry's Therapeutic Treatment Plan. Without adults holding onto their professional boundaries in their work with Harry, he is in danger of his own fantasy view about his reality becoming an actual reality for them to manage and could lead to a breakdown in his behaviour. A note of caution must be raised in relation to ensuring that professional boundaries are maintained by the workers. Not only does this help workers avoid issues of transference and countertransference, but it also helps Harry to understand the meaning of personal responsibility, of understanding and accepting the repercussions of his actions. This could help Harry to see the worker as a separate person from himself, one who is ready to listen to him but not collude with his thoughts and feelings. Should Harry merge with his worker, the worker is in danger of becoming part of Harry's fantasy and will be seen by Harry as part of his traumatic reality. This could inevitably result in over-reactions both from the worker and from Harry.

Final meeting with Harry's key worker and Harry

I met with Harry's key worker six months after the assessment and treatment programme had been put together. I also spent some time with Harry. His key worker told me that because the team had been following the treatment programme for Harry, they were able to be more responsive towards his more complex and at times difficult behaviour. This has resulted in Harry's emotional life strengthening, although there were still numerous times when feelings of panic and rage exploded from him, particularly when he was feeling very anxious.

His capacity to function positively has become stronger, and he is now attending Cadets in the local town and has become a regular member of the team. Importantly, because he was so committed and engaged with the work required of him, he was chosen to take part in the remembrance parade. He was also awarded a first-class medal and has risen to a higher position in his cadet rank. This is a positive outcome for him and has given Harry a more positive sense of his own self.

However, even though Harry's emotional life is stronger, as is his capacity to function since his assessment and Treatment Plan were used, he is still experiencing some difficulties in maintaining friendships with others. Although he now finds the school day more manageable, he continues at times to find managing transitions from one experience of the day to another, quite overwhelming. Harry is moving towards reaching a state of emotional integration (feeling a person in his own right with a sense of self which is developing), but he will continue to find the transition from absolute dependence to inter-dependence difficult and at times painful. The team at the Home has made a good start in working therapeutically with Harry, which he experiences as being real and meaningful to him. Harry experiences a true sense of belonging to the team at the Home. The team recognises that Harry is still deeply emotionally fragile and continues to need a high amount of emotional support and provision from them to help him to feel valued. Although Harry is now approaching 15 years of age, he will continue to need emotional support for the foreseeable future. There is some considerable therapeutic practice to be undertaken with Harry if he is to manage the reality factors of his day-to-day living, but the team have certainly reached the starting point with him, which is a huge achievement.

This case study highlights the positive outcomes for traumatised children and young people when a Needs Led Assessment meets their emotional needs and a treatment programme which workers can put into practice appropriately. However, it is also important that to support them positively, the team of workers develop their own insight and understanding about the more unbearable emotions of the children and young people with whom they work and for them to be aware of how these can impact on themselves. Workers need the opportunity to be reflective about their responses to the events that take place and how these can affect their feelings and their confidence as professionals working with traumatised children and young people.

The case study exemplifies how deeply complex and intense therapeutic work with severely traumatised young people can be for the worker. If we are to prevent young people from requiring serious long-term mental health support, it is crucial that therapeutic work in residential care can identify and reach the 'heart of the matter', namely, the young person's inner world of locked emotions and feelings. The aim is that the young person experiences their stay in the children's Home as one which has given them a secure starting point from which they can continue to emotionally develop their relationship with the outside world. This is not an easy task, but one for which staff require specialist training, consultation, and guidance to learn from. Their work with Harry shows that positive change is possible.

The aim of this chapter has been to demonstrate the importance of the care of children and young people who have been severely traumatised in their early years and the role of therapeutic residential care Homes and treatment centres in helping them to recover and becoming more able to function positively when facing the reality of their day-to-day lives.

Important questions need to be asked: 'What has been the impact of the placement on the lives of children and young people who were originally in care? When they leave their placement, has it been so meaningful for them that they have internalised their stay as a good experience during which time they truly were able to feel that they mattered in a genuine way, and importantly, what had been unbearable emotionally for them when they arrived, had become more bearable in their day-to-day living? Has it helped them to move into the next stage of their lives having established a secure base and sense of their own self as being worthwhile thus enabling them to manage their own reality and become more emotionally thoughtful throughout their lives?

The following two statements, made to me by a young person and an adult, give an insight into their experience of residential care as being positive even though at times painful.

GRACE: A ten-year-old girl who was placed at the community where I was the director of training, came up to me one day and asked me what I did for my work. I explained that my work was to help all those taking care of her and others how to help her and the others with meaning. She said well you are not very good at your work are you? I responded to her, well okay if you think that I am not very good, do let me know what you think it is that I should be doing to make it better. She thought very seriously for some time, then she looked at me intensely and said 'Will you help them [the workers] not just teach them but really help them how to listen to us with their heart and soul, then we shall feel that we are being taken in seriously by them. It emerged that she was a very intelligent girl who had returned from school not having a good day, as she began to act out in the Home where she lived, some workers began to react aggressively towards her and as a result she acted out even more, breaking windows. The comments were an important message from her which I took seriously. I followed this up with the carers trying to help them to understand the importance of responding to traumatised children rather than reacting to them. I saw her again a few weeks later and she said to me 'you are getting better at your job aren't you'. I replied, well thank you that must mean that you are feeling better about yourself' Yes, I am, she replied, and off she skipped.

ALAN: I met Alan at a reunion for adults who had been placed at the Caldecott Community over the past 50 years. He was over 80 years of age when I met him. Alan told me that he loved his times living at the Community, but he had initially been placed at the Mulberry Bush school in Oxfordshire when he was five years old. Because I was surprised him being placed there at such a young age, I asked him if he remembered it? Oh yes, he said I remember Mrs Drysdale (The Director) sitting me on her knee, and playing with me. He went on to elaborate on other good memories of that time at the Bush particularly he enjoyed his opportunities to play with toys and animals. Then he told me that when he was 11 years of age, he was moved over to the Caldecott Community as he had reached adolescence, and 'Miss Leila (then Director of the Caldecott) said to me that she going to help me to have a good education', and similarly as he did with the Mulberry Bush, he continued to tell me stories and memories he held about his time at the Caldecott. I said to him that he did now realise how fortunate he was to have such good memories of his time in the two residential communities. Oh yes, he said to me, because I knew they were always thinking about me. Alan went on to become a successful artist.

Capturing shared memories for a child in care is essential, especially if the child is in a series of foster care placements where they are in danger of feeling invisible and not being thought about, as Alan was. The experience of the poet Lemn Sissay provides a testament to the importance of this and a reminder to residential and foster carers of their role in capturing these memories. Other than Lemn's life record in official reports which he did not have access to as a child, and without access to a mobile phone whilst growing up, few if any photographs exist to verify or record events or milestones in his life as a child. His experience within the care system meant that there was no single individual to remember and bear witness to his life growing up. In his autobiography 'My name is Why?' he wrote,

Memories in care are slippery because there's no one to recall them with as the years pass. In a few months I would be in a different home with a different set of people who had no idea of *this* moment. How could it matter if no one recalls it? Given that staff don't take photographs it was impossible to take something away as a memory. This is how you become invisible. It isn't the lack of photographs that erodes the memory. It is the underlying unkindnesses, which make you feel as though you don't matter enough. This is how to quietly deplete the sense of self-worth deep inside a child's psyche. This is how a child becomes hidden in plain sight. Family is just a set of memories disputed, resolved or recalled between one group of people over a lifetime, isn't it? And if there is no one to care enough to dispute, resolve or recall the memory, then did it happen?
(Sissay, 2020:88)

Summary

This chapter has examined how workers in a therapeutically informed care Home have made a positive impact on the development of a young person through the use of the Needs Led Assessment and Therapeutic Treatment Plans. What has emerged also is that through working with the assessment and Treatment Plans, there has been a change in the teams' insight, understanding, and confidence when they are working with young people with complex histories. Working alongside these young people is not a one-way process, however experienced the worker, and it is important to recognise the potential impact on workers themselves. In trying to understand more about the impact of prolonged trauma on the early lives of children and young people whilst working therapeutically with them, it is inevitable that traumatic episodes which workers themselves have experienced in their lives and their associated anxiety, will surface. Only by being able to reflect and examine behaviour and incidents, and their personal responses to these, will the worker be able to deepen their understanding about the lives of the young people with whom they work, and to respond appropriately, with meaning and integrity. It is crucial that children in need of residential care and treatment find themselves in a position where they have transformed their sense of despair into one of hope during their stay in the Home.

The following poem by Diana Cant captures the emotional chaos and powerlessness experienced by traumatised children when they are unable to communicate.

They push against each other,
Shove forwards, fighting
for his confused attention, why won't they stay still?
Just when he thinks he has them penned
they make a break for it,
spill out
tumble
escape
and he's lost again.

Diana Cant (2021:23) Herding words

Chapter 4

Reparenting traumatised children and young people through adoption

Introduction

An important theme throughout this book has been the impact of trauma on children and young people whose early experiences of emotional abandonment, physical and sexual abuse, and hostility have left them in a position where they often feel attacked by others in the outside world. Their mechanism for survival, consequently, is to attack back. This chapter aims to help post-adoptive parents develop the insight and understanding to enable them to respond appropriately and with sensitivity to the young people they have adopted. Adoptive parents play a critical role in the life of the children and young people and consequently require access to training and guidance to help them recognise what 'difficult to manage behaviour' means. Fundamentally, this is about understanding what it is that the child or young person is trying, but unable, to communicate. They are unable to express the unbearable and unthinkable emotions that they carry with them because of their early trauma as they were not given the opportunity to express themselves in their early years and receive meaningful and real responses from their parental figures. Although the young person can present themselves as being 'fine' on the surface, the slightest stress can cause them to break down, especially where there is a constant fear or anticipation that their new family and adults will repeat their early experiences of trauma. To continue the transition to their new family placement requires guidance and patience. Without appropriate thought and support being given to both the child or young person and the parents, relationships can become increasingly stressful and escalate the acting out of increasing difficult behaviour that the parents are unable to deal with. Without timely and appropriate help and support, the adoption relationship can fall into danger of breaking down.

Since many children and young people of adoptive families are overwhelmed by unbearable and unthinkable anxieties, their relationships with their new families are inevitably shaped by anxieties and fears which have resulted from the original trauma they experienced with their primary carer. The extent and impact of the trauma experienced can result in the child or adolescent being afraid to develop meaningful attachment relationships with the 'new' parent. This fear of commitment to the adoptive parent blocks their maturational development and their developing sense of self, preventing it from strengthening and growing.

DOI: 10.4324/9781003132882-7

To be an adoptive parent can be both a joyful and inspirational task for the parental carers, but also at times overwhelmingly painful for them to manage. Bowlby (1969) wrote that the caregiver's mind offers containment and a secure base which over time become internalised in the child's mind to create mental representations and internal working models. However, where children have found that their caregiver's mind is not safely available to them, for example, in cases of physical abuse, parental drug misuse, or where caregivers themselves have unresolved trauma, children find it difficult to make sense of others or to reflect on, and make their own experiences of the world meaningful. They are left overwhelmed by feelings and thoughts that cannot be organised, and anxieties that cannot be resolved (Schofield, 2005).

The relationships and dynamics in an adoption involving the child, parents, and family members are complex. It is important that adoptive parents can develop and deepen their insight and understanding about the impact that traumatic early experiences can have on the child, and how these experiences can influence their ability to manage the transition to their new family placement. Traumatised children and young people can find the challenges of reality and change too difficult and complex to manage, and so they constantly anticipate that breakdown will occur.

The post-adopted child

Legal adoptions were introduced in England and Wales almost 100 years ago (Adoption of Children's Act 1926). It created a legal fiction (and irrevocable order) which treated a child as if they had been born to the adoptive parents. The new Adoption and Children's Act 2002 came into force in December 2005, replacing the Adoption Act 1976 and the Children's Act 1989, modernising the law regarding adoptive parenting in the UK and international adoption. It also enabled more people to be considered by the adoption agencies as prospective parents. The new Act also placed the needs of the children being adopted above all else. Ofsted (2020) reported that 3,440 children were adopted down 4% (3,590) from previous years and reflected a continued fall since a peak of 5,360 adoptions in 2015.

Adoption is now far more focused on an adopted child being positively influenced in their new family life through building consistent relationships, with the new parents providing the continuity and nurture to help redress the balance in their lives. Effort is made on helping families to think deeply about the complexity of meeting the emotional needs of their adopted child or young person. These emotional needs arise from the fact that the majority of children and adolescents who are being adopted have suffered early trauma including physical, emotional, and often sexual abuse. These experiences are bound in with emotions of panic and rage, which they are not able to think about, and can be acted out towards the new parent in a hostile manner. The cause of this behaviour will occur for a variety of reasons; however, this behaviour can become relentless and exhausting for the new parent to manage, however committed they are towards helping the child or adolescent to develop a strong attachment relationship with them. Without the appropriate guidance and support, it can leave the adoptive parent with strong anxieties and uncertainties about how the relationship can evolve, and about their ability to cope with the child or young person's complex needs within their existing family relationships.

The cases that come to the attention of social and mental health services are so complex that there is a danger of misdiagnoses or superficial labelling, a fact to which Pinto (2019:294) draws attention, reporting that,

> Looked after and adopted children are among the most vulnerable in our society and it is well established that they present with a higher prevalence of mental health problems than children who live with their birth family. In their histories, they frequently have birth parents who have lived chaotic lives, some with mental health problems and substance misuse, and have experienced disruptions of care as well as exposure to neglect and/or abuse. However, often when they try to access mental health services, all their problems are formulated as 'trauma and attachment issues' with lack of data to support these.

The case study presented in this chapter will show how a Needs Led Assessment can shed light on the impact of early trauma and subsequent behaviour providing a deeper understanding about the impact of the trauma. This understanding can enable the adoptive parent to strengthen the child's ability to be able to live with their emotional inner life. Understanding the child's behaviour and what it represents is critical. Without this understanding, both parent and child struggle to understand and manage the child's emotions which erupt as they face any stress in their day-to-day living. The aim is to enable adoptive parents to develop a route to establish a more positive relationship with their adopted child or adolescent. In helping them to meet and provide for the child's unmet early needs, emotional loss, and feelings of abandonment because of their early trauma, the parent can also help them to become more integrated as a person, to express their feelings, think about their anxieties, and steadily mature.

The adopted child presented in the case study has the capacity to display an abundance of charm and friendliness, but his behaviour and level of functioning can become hostile and aggressive when confronted with any stress factor in his life. Both the emotional Needs Led Assessment and Treatment Plan are presented to help the adoptive parent to reach out to the child's unbearable feelings without over-reacting to the child or young person and ultimately to strengthen their confidence and interact more positively with them.

Jimmy

Jimmy lived with his birth family for the first four years of his life. During this period, he was exposed to many disturbing and traumatic episodes including alcoholism, drugs, aggression, violence, constant neglect, and emotional privation. At the age of four years, he was fostered with his two older siblings to whom he was very attached. After one year Jimmy and his sisters were both adopted by different families. The two siblings were together, and Jimmy was on his own not only because he was younger than his siblings, but also because he had been more deeply traumatised by his birth parents. It was felt that he initially required a deeper experience of maternal nurturing from his adoptive mother than his sisters. The result of his early trauma is that he remains a deeply vulnerable and fragmented young person who is emotionally fragile.

Jimmy was adopted at the age of five years through a single-parent adoption. He was experienced by the adoptive mother as functioning on two levels, at times delightful and warm to be with, but at other times prone to fits of fury which were characterised by emotions of panic, rage, and aggression towards her. Unbearable anxiety in the form of panic and rage can erupt without reason in a child who has been traumatised and has no secure attachment. Without help and support, it can become impossible for them to accept personal responsibility for their behaviour.

In contrast, a five-year-old who has experienced a secure attachment with their parent figure, when under pressure, is more likely to express their anxiety in the form of a temper tantrum from which they can explain their reasoning and use it to learn from it as their own sense of self develops and strengthens. The difference is that the anger and frustration expressed by Jimmy are very different and emerge from panic and rage. The former can be thought about, whilst Jimmy's panic and rage are so deeply embedded in his mind that it is difficult and painful to help him communicate his emotions and so the pain remains too unbearable for him to think about.

Jimmy is now 12 years of age and has been with the adoptive mother for the past 6 years. The adoptive mother and her wider family remain totally committed to Jimmy and his placement with her, but she is also deeply concerned about his capacity to function appropriately during his journey into adolescence. Any stress factor in his day-to-day living leads to him becoming socially and emotionally isolated. Although he remains deeply attached and absolutely dependent on his mother, he is finding it almost impossible to be separated from her, and he continues to experience the outside world as being almost impossible to manage.

I met Jimmy once briefly after I had met the adoptive mother; I experienced him as a delightful young person but who was also emotionally fragile. In discussion with the mother, the three areas of the emotional Needs Led Assessment programme which needed to be discussed about Jimmy were as follows:

1 Containing emotion, anxiety, anger, and stress.
2 Self-esteem and self-preservation.
3 Separation and loss, and managing transitions.

1   Containing emotion, anxiety, anger, and stress

Since his adoption, Jimmy's behaviour fluctuates between presenting himself as being charming and engaging, but the slightest stress factor in his day-to-day living results in aggressive and violent episodes which causes him to behave destructively or self-destructively. This can be very difficult and painful for his adoptive mother to manage.

Although she has been able to manage such episodes of acting out, at times it had been very painful for her to hold onto Jimmy without over-reacting to his behaviour negatively. Nevertheless, after a period of time of him living with his new mother in her home, he became more able to apologise for his behaviour. Jimmy has a fragile sense of self, and he cannot cope with any sense of loss in his day-to-day living. An example of this is his fears and worries that his mother may die or disappear when he is not with her. Although he has developed a strong attachment to his adoptive mother, he has not been able to develop a sense of individuality and personal development. Since he has suffered such intense early trauma, he still needs to remain absolutely dependent on her because he cannot yet cope with managing himself. Jimmy's sense of self is emotionally raw, and he finds it very difficult to manage separation and loss. Where he experiences times in the outside world as traumatic, the sadness that he feels is overwhelming. This brings up emotions which are a result of his early traumas. This can result in feelings of emotional abandonment and of being attacked by others. It makes him think that he needs to control the environment that he is living in because he is afraid of losing everything he loves, but at the same time, it can result in him becoming overwhelmed with feelings of despair and sadness which can take him back to his inner feelings of emotional isolation.

Although Jimmy is now far more approachable at his times of stress than when he was originally adopted, he still requires a high degree of emotional support when he ceases to function. He does, however, have some emotional resources on which he is able to draw. There are certain circumstances in his day-to-day living when he finds the pressure of meeting the challenges which occur in certain aspects of his daily living impossible and unbearable to manage. Jimmy is functioning at the level of a fragmented/archipelago child. There are parts of the day when he is able to function well, but the slightest stress factor or anxiety results in him ceasing to function. He has formed a meaningful attachment with his adoptive mother. Nevertheless, because he is so emotionally fragile, when under stress, he becomes in danger of disintegrating, returning to a state where his anger and overwhelming anxiety control him, effecting his behaviour.

Therapeutic Treatment Plan

Jimmy's capacity to function is limited, and he can easily become overwhelmed with anxiety and fear which block his capacity to function. When he feels hopeless and helpless about his own sense of self, and despair about life, he shuts down, withdrawing into himself and goes to his bedroom. It is important to realise this behaviour for what it represents and that because of Jimmy's early traumatic experiences, he gave up any hope of feeling positive about his own purpose in living. It was only when he was being taken care of by his older sisters and now by his adoptive mother, that he feels more emotionally contained and can function. However, he is not yet ready to function positively in his own world as an individual with his own sense of purpose and individuality.

To help him move towards feeling stronger with a growing belief in his developing sense of self, the following points are important:

1 Acknowledge his feelings of anxiety and fear and let him know that you are aware and understand how painful taking risks can be for him at times. Try to help him to communicate what it is that he is afraid will happen to him, reassuring him that you will be supporting him through his painful times.

2 Help him to realise that you are aware that when he experiences situations in the outside world which make him feel angry and sad, it can feel too much for him because perhaps it reminds him of when he felt very sad and lost as a small child. Explain that it is a very different world that he is living in now, and that you want to help him manage, and tackle the challenges he is faced with currently.

2 Self-esteem and self-preservation

Self-esteem

Jimmy believes that anything he attempts in life will be catastrophic, and anything good and positive could break down. He feels isolated in his day-to-day living with little or no peer support from friends. He does not yet feel ready or secure enough to integrate himself into a peer group or create friendships with others. Jimmy has little self-esteem and at times shows no capacity to survive his unbearable feelings. Instead, he idealises himself and sees himself as a 'hero' who is out to save the world. This represents the part of Jimmy which he feels needs protecting by his carers.

It is important to recognise that he cannot manage ambivalence and is unable to express doubts and uncertainty about his current situation and any conflicts, nor is he able to psychologically contain positive and negative feelings. Instead, he seeks situations that he can idealise, looking for a perfect solution, yet when feelings of anxiety and stress overwhelm him, he denigrates his current situation and sees his experience as being unworkable, and so he tries to extinguish it, either by isolating himself or becoming aggressive and attacking others.

Self-preservation

Jimmy cannot take care of himself physically, nor can he value himself. This is most likely because he does not have any sense of enjoying and valuing any good experience he receives. Even when good experiences have occurred, they could not be perceived as a worthwhile experience for him. Jimmy's self-esteem and lack of value in himself are so intense that he is unable to be positive about what he has experienced. In this category as before, Jimmy is a fragmented/

archipelago child with bits and pieces of positive aspects of his life, but which can very easily break down and once again become negative responses.

Therapeutic Treatment Plan

When Jimmy's self-esteem weakens, his sense of despair and hopelessness come to the fore, and he feels that he cannot achieve anything. His sense of self feels threatened, and he attempts to destroy anything that felt positive in his life. His fear of managing reality and the challenges of the outside world are foremost in his thinking, and he ceases to try to function in external reality. This results in him falling into himself and 'hiding away' both psychologically and physically. To help his parent see him through this painful episode, the following point should be thought about:

- Help Jimmy to realise that you understand that managing stress is difficult for him and give him coping mechanisms to manage them. Help him to identify what his main fears and anxieties are and how they affect him.
- Help him to identify the main areas of his day-to-day living which produces powerful emotions in him that he needs to face, identify, and focus on the two areas of day-to-day living situations he needs most help with, and together write a plan as to how you can help him manage these.
- Jimmy is confused about parenting styles because he was so traumatised by his birth parent and his mind still feels that these early experiences will re-occur, even though the parenting style of his adopted parent is very different and positive. Although he desires her nurturing and responsiveness, he cannot believe that it will continue if his behaviour is difficult, and so expects hostility, emotional abandonment, and negative reactivity from her. He cannot believe that a good experience will continue regardless of his behaviour.
- Jimmy requires support and help to be able to distinguish between fantasy and reality. When he is feeling emotionally fragile, his imagination takes over, and he believes that terrible things will happen, and becomes the basis for his reality. He requires his mother or other carers to help him to be more realistic about his situation, which is more independent in his mind.

Help him to see that reality can become more bearable and acceptable so that he can work at it with their help.

3 Separation and loss, and managing transitions

Jimmy did not experience an early maternal experience from which he was able to make the natural transition from absolute dependence from his mother, through to a sense of inter-dependence and individuality to form the basis of his maturational development. In contrast, because his adoptive mother is responding to him in a very nurturing and caring manner, Jimmy feels the need to regress to an infantile stage because he finds the transition from infancy to latency and adolescence impossible to manage. Although he is now 12 years of age, there remains a part of Jimmy in his internal world which remains feeling like a two-to three-year-old. It is important that both aspects are responded to by his mother without him regressing back to functioning like a two- to three-year-old. Jimmy is a very vulnerable young person, and this needs to be recognised.

Therapeutic Treatment Plan

The following points are important in helping Jimmy to develop greater confidence in being separated, and in beginning to manage the process of transition:

- Help Jimmy to communicate his fears and anxieties about separating from his adopted mother. Ask him what he could take with him to help his transition to school or another change of territory. Help him to realise that you continue to hold him in your mind, thinking about him when he is not there with you.
- Try to identify what you could provide Jimmy with when he returns from school at the end of the day. By creating a space for you and him to discuss the positive and negative aspects of his day, you will be providing a stepping stone, helping him with the process of transition until he can start to think about the day himself.

Jimmy is a very emotionally fragile young person who was severely traumatised in his early years. Finding the starting point to help him manage and value himself in his new family is complicated. However, because the adoptive mother is so committed to responding and providing for his previous unmet emotional needs, there is a very strong possibility that in time she will be able to find the appropriate starting point to help him to become more emotionally integrated being able to think through his own feelings and face the reality of managing his own life.

The next phase is for me to visit Jimmy's mother and go through the Needs Led Assessment and Therapeutic Treatment programme with her and discuss how the Treatment Plan can be implemented.

My visit with Jimmy and his mother

I visited Jimmy's mother three times, once to go through the assessment and Treatment Plan with her, the other to spend a short period of time with both Jimmy and her together, and finally to get her feedback about how she found the Treatment Plan. On reading the assessment and Treatment Plan, she agreed that it did portray how she experienced working and living with Jimmy.

Currently, Jimmy is having a difficult time and is unable to manage in the educational setting. Not only is he emotionally fragile, but also the COVID pandemic has made him feel even more isolated and he has retreated into himself, cutting himself off from the outside world. He says that he is afraid of leaving his mother because he fears that she may have an accident or die. He is absolutely dependent and deeply worried about losing her. I suggested to him that perhaps this was because he thought badly of himself at times and was afraid that he would not be able to manage his day-to-day living without her being there. He told me that he felt there were a lot of things wrong with him and that he did not know where to begin. I responded that perhaps he and his mother could work together towards finding a new starting point when managing his daily life.

I visited again a few weeks later for a short period to spend some more time with them. Jimmy was very anxious about me coming to see them and was in his room when I arrived. His mother explained to me that when he panicked, he would take to his room until he felt that he could manage his world again. He came down after a few minutes, and it seemed that he was pleased to see me, smiling as we sat down to he began to speak. Jimmy's placement in his current school had broken down, and he did not want to return. He told me that he no longer felt that there was a place for him in his old school, mainly because he had been out of school and at home for a few months because of the COVID pandemic which had brought back his feelings of emotional isolation which he could not let go. However, there had been a subsequent meeting and he was told that he could be changed to a school where he felt he would be happier. I pointed out that this could be a new starting point for him, but that we all need to work hard at a starting point to ensure that we can carry on working through difficult periods in our lives whilst also valuing the positive and fulfilling moments in our day-to-day living. He thought that would be a good idea to work on.

I found the time I spent with Jimmy and his mother interesting, thought-provoking, and emotionally moving. The mother is totally committed to helping Jimmy through his difficulties and to be able to continue functioning more positively throughout his day-to-day living. However, it is a difficult task for her because he was traumatised in his infantile years, although he is now 12 years old, and has become dependent on her for his emotional needs, ones left over from his infancy. Donald Winnicott (1971:60) defined the concept of an infant being 'absolutely dependent' on their primary carer as being crucial, a key stepping stone until they are able to make the transition through to inter-dependence that enables them to manage the transition from infancy to latency, and towards adolescent development in their lives. Jimmy did not experience such with his birth mother, and currently, he does not believe that he exists at all without his adoptive mother being there for him continually.

There are two concepts of the Treatment Plan which may help her to help Jimmy to move forward having developed a greater sense of hope about himself in his future life.

- Transference and countertransference
- Managing transitions

1 Transference and Countertransference

Transference describes the process through which the child transfers onto the carer, feelings and ideas that belong to previous experiences in their lives, which for Jimmy include both positive and traumatic experiences. The outcome is that at times he will be able to function like a 12-year-old, but other times, he will present the emotional needs of an infant who wants constant emotional preoccupation from his mother. The panic and fear he experiences when he is overwhelmed with anxiety will be projected onto his adoptive mother, which she will experience as quite overwhelming at times.

Countertransference represents the feelings and responses of the worker or parent, which are affected by the child's unbearable emotions being projected onto them by the child or young person producing different reactions from them. Although Jimmy's needs have been so demanding at times on her, through his mother's devotion to him, he is slowly being able to hold on to unbearable feelings and start to communicate them both verbally and symbolically. Understanding the transference and countertransference feelings that emerge could be helpful to enable them to arrive at a new starting point together.

2 Managing transitions

Jimmy finds change and new beginnings difficult to manage. He has only survived his fears and anxieties by building up a false self which presents himself as being excited when his inner uncertainties and anxieties haunt him, leading to breakdown at a later stage. To help him realise and accept that transitions are not always easy, and to support him to make it more manageable, it is important to help him express his fears and anxieties.

Help him to become aware that you are there and able to discuss these with him. This may help him to achieve a sense of hope about the next stage of his life becoming more acceptable and important than the previous. Currently, Jimmy is dependent on his mother as a transitional object, but if Jimmy can adopt an alternative transitional object as described by Winnicott (1971:5), one that represents the meaning of his relationship with his mother, this may help to prevent him from worrying that she may not be there whilst he is engaged in any new environment such as going to school. The transitional object acts as a reminder that his mother is still thinking about him.

I met with Jimmy's mother a few months later to discuss with her how she had found being with Jimmy after the assessment and Treatment Plan programme and if she was aware of any changes in his view of himself as a person. By this time, Jimmy had started at a new school. However, he found the experience difficult, and because he had not been able to attend school earlier because of COVID, he felt emotionally isolated from other children in his class. He found the experience of being a part of group difficult to sustain and the fact that he could not take part in group activities not only reinforced his isolation, but also increased his fear of being separated from his adoptive mother. Nevertheless, with support from the post-adoption team and hard work on the mother's side, they have now been able to place Jimmy into a pupil referral unit for three months to prepare him to integrate into an alternative school setting later in the year.

I asked his mother what she felt she had gained from her introduction to Needs Led Assessment programme and Treatment Plan. She reflected that although he is more positive about the new school placement, she is only too aware of his anxieties and how the slightest difficulty he experiences in the school could immediately take him backwards. To help Jimmy to separate from her, she has given him a very special stone that he is very attached to and that he takes with him each day and keeps in a safe place in his pocket. The message for Jimmy is that he can touch the stone whenever he wishes, and in doing so, he is reminded that he remains in the mind of his mother whilst he is in school.

She found that having a deeper understanding about Jimmy had helped her to be far more insightful into his behaviour. Jimmy now talks about the importance of 'finding a new starting point' in his daily living experiences and being able to manage them more positively. He is a very complex young person having been so traumatised at an early stage of his development, but if he is to arrive at, and maintain the road to his recovery, it is crucial that the mother can afford to 'bear the unbearable' in his day-to-day living experiences. This could result in the fragmented aspects of his emotional life starting to come together, creating a more emotionally integrated young person who is becoming more positive about the experiences in his day-to-day living.

My personal reflection

I have found the experience of spending time with Jimmy and his mother both moving and emotional. Children who have been traumatised in their early years find the opportunity of maintaining a meaningful attachment with adults difficult, complex, and painful. However, because his mother is totally committed in helping him to feel better about himself and because he is also seeing a child psychotherapist whom he enjoys seeing, he is in a position where with their support and his understanding, he knows that he is thought about by them. Jimmy is developing the capacity to bear the most unbearable aspects of his everyday living, slowly working towards finding a new starting point in his life.

Conclusion

This chapter has tried to highlight the importance of the underlying commitment which is needed from adoptive parents when they are parenting children and young people who have been severely traumatised in their early years before they were adopted. If the child is to reach the capacity to trust others in their lives, they require parents who can 'bear the unbearable' when some of the most unbearable feeling and emotions start to emerge from the child and is thrown back at the parent. If their internal emotional world can be understood and responded to with meaning and sincerity, it can result in the child feeling that they really do matter as a person who can be an individual in their own right. If they do not understand why they are feeling as they do, how can the parent make any decisions about their lives which does not link into the child's own internal world?

I am reminded of a statement the psychoanalyst and paediatrician Dr Donald Winnicott made to me many years ago when he was a consultant to a therapeutic community for adolescents at which I worked. I wanted his advice about a teenage boy I was working with building a model village. Some days the village was alive, trees were growing, with busy shops and where people were speaking to each other. The next day, the village had died, the trees stopped growing, and nobody was living there. I told Dr Winnicott that I did not quite understand what he was trying to communicate to me through his play. He observed the village quietly and deeply, and after a few minutes, he looked back at me and said 'do you know what my dear, neither do I'. I was rather surprised that such an eminent psychiatrist did not know what the boy was trying to communicate in his building and destruction of the model village. Then, he said to me, 'but my dear Christine carry on not knowing and one day the true meaning will emerge from him with meaning and sincerity. If one feels that they have to know all the time, often they do not know at all. But if they can afford to live with not knowing, the real knowing will emerge with meaning. So, my dear carry on not knowing and the truth will arrive'. I followed his advice, and it was true, in time the boy was able to tell me that he felt dead inside himself at times. And we worked from there.

Finally, as Jimmy starts to feel more real and alive because his adoptive mother has been able to live alongside his most unbearable emotional moments and survive, he is beginning to communicate about finding a new starting point in his life. As he starts to feel more real as an individual, he is beginning to think about himself and to manage reality with enthusiasm and a sense of belief in himself. It is an arduous task for parents, carers, and other workers involved with adopted children, but crucial if we are to help them to become a person in their own right, with a view of the world that is manageable and workable. It is a long-term task which must be thought of not just in terms of the here and now, but in terms of the young person's life and future. With patience and understanding, an adoptive parent can make it possible for an adopted young person who has been as overwhelmed with unbearable pain, loss, and isolation as has Jimmy, to see that change is possible and that they can move forward feeling better about themselves both in their day-to-day living and with their future.

Twelve months later, Jimmy continues to persevere through difficult and painful moments in his day-to-day living. He is now more able to think about his emotions, which are unbearable at times, but this is something that he was not able to achieve in the early days of his adoption. His mother continues to live through his struggles with him, which can also be rather painful for her at times. However, her emotional commitment towards Jimmy and his future development is hopeful, and most sincere on her part. She recognises that when a child was so traumatised in their early life as Jimmy, it is inevitable that this will have an impact on their future development. We cannot idealise what occurs, but if Jimmy continues to make the best of what he has gained through this relationship, this will be a huge achievement for both of them. I am most grateful and honoured to have been able to spend some time working with Jimmy and his mother.

Chapter 5

Preparing traumatised children and adolescents for long-term foster placement

Introduction

The complexities for adoptive parents and residential workers when they are caring for children and young people who have been so deeply traumatised by both the abusive and hostile experiences they have endured, and the painful and difficult process of forming positive attachment relationships with adult carers, are evident. This chapter explores the experiences of both the child and the foster parents in managing the transition from abusive family settings to ones where parent figures are more focused on positive family relationships. In working with carers and workers, it has become clear that both recognise the need to gain a deeper insight and understanding about meeting the emotional needs of traumatised children and young people and how this can influence their response to their new family experience. Over 53,400 children are fostered in the UK (Narey and Owers, 2018). In addition to early experiences of trauma, neglect, and abuse, the reported data shows that the majority of children in foster care are male (54%), white (76%), and over the age of 10 (60%) with only 18% aged 4 and under (2018:17–18).

It is important that foster parents have an in-depth understanding of the child that they have agreed to foster. Many children who are placed in foster care by social services carry early childhood experiences of trauma with their birth family and an internal world fraught with feelings of uncertainty, insecurity, fear, and panic. The legacy of these early experiences leaves them both insecure and uncertain about their relationship with their new family. Although they can attach to their new foster parents, it may be very difficult for them to maintain and develop positive attachment relationships with them. The child's experiences of their previous parents were ones of abuse towards them, and so their expectations are inevitable that these same experiences will re-occur in their new family placement. Their internal world of locked-away emotions could surface when the new foster parents try to manage behaviours with firm, loving boundaries, which the child or young person sees as attacking and hostile, mirroring the abusive parents they had in their previous family life. This could result in them acting out destructively towards the foster parents, or self-destructively towards themselves, putting the placement in danger of breaking down. The compulsion to repeat past traumatic experiences

DOI: 10.4324/9781003132882-8

is overwhelming and becomes paramount in the child's mind. These repressed unbearable emotions that arise out of their earlier trauma critically spill over into their interactions with their foster parents who find the child difficult to manage and emotionally contain. Humphreys *et al.* (2018:821) provide evidence that early fostering of children and young people who have experienced severe deprivation and reduced time in institutional care has a significant impact on adaptive functioning.

It is acknowledged that fostering a traumatised child is generally more complex and difficult than previously recognised, particularly when they are helping and supporting them to develop emotionally and cognitively. This view is supported by Narey and Owers (2018:91), who report in their review, that

> The degree of developmental trauma experienced by children in the looked after system means they often require very intensive developmental re-parenting. Deficits and damage caused by early poor parenting means that, in order to heal and catch up, children require to be parented as much younger children.

It is essential that foster carers are given adequate information prior to the child coming into their homes to enable them to prepare how to care and manage them. The same applies to the child themselves. Regulation 11 requires that the child is properly prepared for a placement with information about the carers, their family and the carers' home, day-to-day care, and routines before the first meeting (including seeing video messages and scenes of their bedroom and learning about some basic house rules) (Narey and Owers, 2018:78).

Successful foster placements are characterised as 'providing a safe and nurturing environment with appropriate support and encouragement for the child or young person to improve their confidence and self-esteem about themselves and their day-to-day living' (Cambrian Care Group, 2022). Importantly, 'placing children into families following severe deprivation increases the likelihood of adaptive functioning in early adolescence' (Humphreys *et al.*, 2018:811).

Providing emotionally significant foster placements for traumatised children and young people is critical, however the question must be asked: where do we find the starting point for them? How can we identify what it is they really need and require from the foster parents if they are to allow themselves to feel valued and emotionally contained by them, to the extent that they can internalise their experience with the family, as one from which they genuinely feel valued and accepted with such certainty about themselves? Children and young people able to integrate into their new family setting will be able to establish a secure base within themselves which will provide them with a new starting point in their lives, and importantly, it will help them to develop and strengthen their own sense of self.

This chapter will present two case studies. The first case study is of Jess and highlights the care and treatment which this young person needs to enable her to relate to and attach to carers in new family placement. The Needs Led Assessment and Treatment Plan programme carried out within a residential care setting can provide foster carers with the insight and understanding about the child or young person's emotional and maturational development to help them evolve and prepare for a foster family placement.

Case study 2 will investigate the demands on foster carers who care for a severely traumatised child or adolescent, and their capacity to bear the unbearable feelings expressed by the child when they are caring for them.

Case study: Jess

Background

Jess was eight years old when she was placed into foster care. She spent the first eight years of her life in a very dysfunctional family with seven brothers and sisters; a mother who was deeply depressed with a very low cognitive ability and a history of domestic abuse, drug dependency, and little energy or ability to emotionally nurture her children. In addition to this, there was evidence of aggressive behaviour from the father towards Jess. The only members of the family to whom she was attached were one or two of her brothers and sisters.

The case history from the social worker stated that all the children suffered from long-term neglect which had caused harm to their emotional and physical wellbeing. Eventually, all the children were placed into foster placements. Jess experienced three foster placements in an 18-month period, but each broke down because of her difficult behaviour. In one of the placements, she was violent and physically aggressive towards the foster parents, and in the second, her aggression and violence were so powerful that the foster carer became afraid of her. Although Jess experienced greater stability initially in the third placement, the aggressive and violent aspects of her behaviour resulted in Jess trying to push the foster carer down the stairs. In addition, she was also very envious of the foster parents' own child whom she could not prevent herself from constantly watching and standing outside the child's bedroom door. All these elements of her behaviour resulted in the placement breaking down.

Eventually at the age of ten, Jess was placed in a residential setting which specialised in preparing children for successful long-term fostering. It was decided that to support this, a Needs Led Assessment and Treatment Plan should be written that would help the team manage Jess in a more positive way and help Jess work through aspects of her behaviour that she found difficult to manage.

Needs Led Assessment and Therapeutic Treatment Plan

The Needs Led Assessment programme and Treatment Plan carried out identified four key areas from the potential seven categories available:

- Boundaries, merging and functioning.
- Self-esteem and self-preservation.
- Communication.
- Play.

1 Boundaries, merging and functioning

The main focus in this category is that the child should have the capacity to hold onto boundaries and carry a sense of personal responsibility for their behaviour when they are being difficult and challenging in their day-to-day living situation. Children whose early traumas have fragmented their personality and sense of self find it difficult, and at times impossible, to hold onto boundaries because they hold an expectation that external reality is there to attack them. This makes them feel that they have to attack back.

With appropriate support from the residential team, Jess can hold onto boundaries, but she finds it very difficult to deal with stressful factors, becoming emotionally isolated and in danger of breaking down. Since Jess's sense of self is emotionally fragile most of the time, she finds it very difficult to be positive about her day-to-day living experiences. This is because she does not believe that she is worthy of a positive experience in her life and has little value on her own sense of self. Jess can hold onto boundaries when their importance is explained to her by the workers. The difficulty for Jess is that she is so emotionally fragile that when others over-react to her, she becomes afraid that she is being attacked, seeing it as a repetition of earlier traumatic experiences in her life. This can result in her breaking through the boundaries and not keeping to the rules. However, the team are hopeful for her and inform me that when responded to appropriately, she has the capacity to become more reflective about her behaviour and is beginning to accept personal responsibility for her difficult actions when they occur.

2 Self-esteem and self-preservation

Jess's way of dealing with stressful times is for her to withdraw from others and to self-isolate. Her view of herself is very low. Her chronological age at times comes over to the workers as being that of a two-year-old who needs constant reassurance from others. She needs to feel that she is consistently being held in the mind of those caring for her with empathic thoughts and responsiveness from them. This is an emotion that she did not receive in her early years. Consequently, she finds becoming attached to adults in her relationships difficult and at times unbearable to hold onto. This can result in Jess feeling emotionally attacked by others, and she can attack back as a reaction to the hurt and pain she carries in her internal world.

3 Communication and play

The two separate areas of communication and play have been brought together in this section as it's seen that one is able to help the development of the other.

Jess has been left with a range of thoughts and emotions that she is not yet ready to communicate verbally. However, she does find playing at a symbolic level helpful and creative for her. The writing of poetry and songs is her way of expressing thoughts and feelings that she is not able to express verbally. The use of performing arts is crucial as it helps her to continue to explore and develop her own sense of self in a positive way.

Therapeutic Treatment Plan

- It is important that Jess feels constantly held in the mind of those responsible for her.
- Work needs to be done to help Jess manage external reality and understand how her own inner fears and anxieties influence her capacity to meet the needs and demands of the outside world, at times making it more difficult for her to think consistently about her actions.
- Be aware of the level of Jess's low self-esteem and how that can influence her behaviour and her capacity to function positively.
- Understanding the impact of transference and countertransference on Jess's relationships through attachment with others.

1   Held in mind

The concept of being 'held in mind' by their carer is critical to children who have suffered early trauma. They need to know that their carer is constantly thinking of them. Where an infant misses out on fundamental infantile experiences where they did not feel thought about, responded to, and emotionally contained, they are unable to build up functioning internal controls and cannot regulate their emotions. Children who do not feel safe in infancy have trouble regulating their moods and emotional responses as they grow older (van der Kolk, 2014), leading them to believe that their anxieties and uncertainties cannot be expressed. To compensate for this, they either build up a 'false self' to protect themselves from their unbearable feelings and emotions, or start to act out their panic and rage, often aggressively, towards others.

Helping Jess believe that she is held in mind and that she really does exist as a person in her own right is critical. She needs to understand and believe that her key worker is in touch with her own internalised thoughts and the feelings of disbelief that she carries about in relation to her own sense of self. It is important that her key worker is able to help Jess to think about her day and identify the areas that could help her to communicate her own anxieties and fears of the outside world. She needs to be helped to realise that her key worker will be thinking about her throughout her day. When she returns from school, ensure that her key worker spends some quiet time with her to ask about the positive and negative aspects of her day. Think about a special drink or food that would always be there for Jess at specific times of the day. This should help her to truly believe that she is held in the mind of her key worker in a positive way.

2   Self-esteem and self-preservation

If a child has no sense of self-esteem, they are often unable to take care of themselves. Their level of despair is so great they become overwhelmed by a sense of self-reprisal, and they can act out destructively or self-destructively or else self-isolate themselves from others.

In helping Jess to feel more emotionally contained, the key worker will help her to work towards developing a stronger view of herself as a person who matters.

3   Managing internal and external reality factors in her day-to-day living

As Jess has been subjected to traumatic experiences in her early life, her internal world of painful memories will be laden with emotions of anxiety and despair. This will influence how she relates to external reality and managing the pressures that emerge. She requires her workers to be in touch with her when she is overwhelmed by her own anxieties, responding to her fears and uncertainties and asking her whether they can do anything to help her to feel better about herself. The more she can communicate how she feels, the more she will move towards developing the strength required to take on board the challenges of the reality factors she has to face in her life.

Summary

Jess is functioning at the level of a fragmented/archipelago child. The result of her early trauma has left her feeling trapped in her own internal world, with a range of thoughts and emotions that she is not yet ready to communicate verbally. At times, she can become overwhelmed by her emotions and has to isolate herself from others because she fears reacting aggressively towards them and the repercussions that follow. This explains why she finds attachment relationships difficult to sustain. To survive, she has built up a 'false self' to protect herself from some of her own panic, rage, and despair. Importantly, the team feel that she is slowly starting to develop a sense of hope about her future rather than the constant despair she exhibited in the beginning, and recognise that she will remain emotionally fragile for some time until her sense of self has strengthened.

To help understand how living alongside Jess impacts on the internal world of the workers, I spent a full day working as a part of the team in the home where Jess is placed.

A day in the life of Jess

I visited the Home to work as a member of the team for the day. Although Jess had told her worker that she wanted to see me, when I arrived, I found that she was not ready to come down but preferred to stay in her room. Eventually, she came back down to watch the television and I went over to sit with her and asked if she remembered me as I had spoken to her previously asking for permission to use her case in my forthcoming book. She did agree for which I was most grateful, and also chose the name to use when discussing her case. She then asked me if I would like to watch her dance, and I replied that I would be delighted to do so. I went to her room with Jess and a worker to whom she was attached. She played music which was deep and powerful, and for 15 minutes, she danced beautifully with a very intense movement and did not stop until the music had ceased. I congratulated her and said that I had thoroughly enjoyed watching her dance. I said that it seemed to me that her dancing was her way of expressing some of the emotions, which felt trapped inside her and which she was not able to communicate verbally. She nodded and said that it was right. There were feelings inside her which she did not wish to talk about yet.

After we had gone for a walk and had lunch with another child and the team, Jess began to watch the television. She was most interested and explained to me that the film she was watching was about evil trying to stop good things happening, and you had to fight against it to prevent them from winning. I then asked if she would like to make up a story about that, with myself and she said that she would very much. I began telling the story about three farming families who decided to go for a walk. After a few minutes, Jess then took over the story by telling how that journey became hazardous and dangerous for the families. They became separated from each other, and fell into territories with evil creatures trying to prevent them from finding their way back home. Eventually, Jess was able to present how all three families were able to find a way home and beat the terror of the evil creatures. I then completed the story by telling how they were able to come together and celebrate their journey its dangers and successes. Jess spoke for about 20 minutes; she was so involved in the story. I found the time we spent together telling the story (mainly by Jess) moving and insightful. The difficulties, fears, and challenges the families had to endure when finding their way home represented Jess's view of her own life. Before I left the Home after having been there for several hours, I went back to Jess and told her that I was having to leave now, but that I wanted to say goodbye to her and thank her for such an enjoyable day in the Home, and being able to spend some time with her. We had spoken at times about her wanting a new family who she could live with, even though the previous ones had not been too successful. Her last statement to me as she curled up in her chair was:

> I do feel happy and secure in the home, and I know that now is not the right time for me to have a new family, but I truly hope that in time there will be a new family who would want to give me a new life.

I found my day with Jess and the team in her Home deeply thought-provoking, emotionally moving, and quite inspirational. It made me realise how crucial it is that both the residential workers and foster carers are able to recognise the impact the child or young person's emotional fragility had on their relationship with them as substitute parents, following the trauma they experienced in their own families.

I have concluded that foster carers need specialist support if they are to allow a child or young person's sense of self to strengthen and develop whilst they are placed with them.

The task is for the young person to start to believe that their new family experience can be internalised as a fresh and more solid starting point in their life, moving beyond the trauma they experienced in their previous family.

Specialist support should focus on enabling foster parents to understand more about the painful emotions the child or young person carries with them as a result of their previous unsuccessful placements, either from their primary family or with alternative ones. These can emerge during stressful situations within their current family, occurring because they are overwhelmed with unbearable thoughts and feelings carried from their previous placements. Managing this is not an easy task for foster parents, but crucial if they are to help the child or young person to work through some of their most painful emotions concerning their relationship with external reality when their own internal world is flooded with unbearable feelings that they do not yet feel emotionally secure enough to be able to think about.

Case study: examining the experience of foster parents and social workers

To understand the areas of anxiety and uncertainty foster carers have to endure when they were going through difficult periods with the foster child's behaviour, I met with four individuals with thorough knowledge of the care system. The group comprised two experienced foster carers Tom and Ann, willing to talk about the complexity of the emotions and experiences of fostering children and young people, and two social workers who have supported a number of foster carers through emotionally painful and difficult times arising from the foster child's behaviour in their family environment. I felt it was important that the social workers who supported the foster carers were present at our discussion, both to reassure them and to act as a point of reference should the need arise. It was agreed by the foster parents that any confidential information which arose in our discussion would not be reported within this chapter. Our discussion was framed by four key questions which were sent to them prior to our meeting to allow them time to reflect.

The first question asked them to identify the key areas of support and training required for a foster parent if they were to achieve a deeper and more significant understanding and insight about the appropriate responses required from them when a child or young person ceased to function and could not manage reality.

Both Tom and Ann explained that at times they had found it difficult to manage their own expectations of the foster child whilst they were living within the dynamics of their own families and identify the impact this had on them. However, they did realise that their expectations of the child arose from their role as substitute parents. With support from their social workers, they came to realise that their expectations of the foster children at times were too high and in fact unachievable. They realised that it was the emotional growth and learning that they themselves had developed as foster parents which helped them to respond appropriately to the child or young person during times of difficult and erratic behaviour. It was the interaction during these times which resulted in the child developing a more significant and meaningful attachment relationship with their foster parents, and as one of the foster parents observed,

> Fostering any child is always an evolving practice, every child is different and reacts to different situations completely differently. It takes time to get to know your foster children and what works best for them

> (Tom)

They were clear that foster parents need to have ongoing support and consultation during which time they are given the space to reflect on the difficulties in parenting children and young people who constantly expect negative and hostile reactions from their parental figures. Having the opportunity to examine how that affected them and influenced their relationship with the child or young person was seen to be very important. They acknowledged that reflective practice, discussions, and guidance by social workers have helped them to be more thoughtful about their practice and more insightful about the way they dealt with difficult and potentially destructive behaviours in the children and young people that they fostered.

The second question centred on how foster parents managed the child's or young person's complex behaviour.

The key themes that emerged from the discussion were that of being able to anticipate and intervene appropriately. Both Tom and Ann told me that being able to identify the behaviours when they were emerging, and being given some possible ways to help deal with them would be most important for the child's or young person's personal maturation in their foster home. In answer to the question, Ann reflected,

> Some of the behaviours we have had to deal with have been very hard for us, but we fully understand the reason behind them and their troubled start in life. We can now manage these behaviours naturally and is a part of our lives and theirs. It is only when our placement goes on respite, that we actually sit back and note how much work monitoring on a daily basis we carry out.

Foster parents do require some insight and understanding as to how they can identify the meaning of the foster child's behaviour and how they can best intervene before they become too destructive towards themselves and others.

The third question explored whether foster parents were aware of the point at which the child or young person started to attach and become dependent on their new family, and whether they were aware of the positive and negative emotions, which could arise in both themselves as parents and the child or young person.

Both Tom and Ann were familiar with the period of the child settling in, the 'lull before the storm' at which point the child's behaviour begins to escalate. This could be difficult and painful for them to understand and manage. The point at which the child begins to attach themselves to the adult carers brings out a number of anxieties and insecurities about trusting others, because their earlier traumas have left them in fear of being re-traumatised.

A child who has experienced numerous traumatic experiences in their early years both emotionally and physically finds attaching to parental figures they are fostered with complex and difficult. Their expectations are that the original experiences of emotional abandonment, abuse, and hostility will be recreated in their new family environment. As a result of their early trauma, their sense of self can be very fragile and 'their internal working model and sense of self is less positive than the experiences of the child who is securely attached' (Howe, 2011:190). Before they can reach the stage of becoming securely attached to the foster parents, the foster parents require appropriate training and guidance to clarify how they can provide emotional and practical support for the child. This understanding will help strengthen the child's ability and emotional strength that will enable them to live alongside the day-to-day reality of their lives and, importantly, will help the child to begin the process of achieving a meaningful attachment with the foster parents.

The fourth question asked foster parents to identify specific areas or concepts that they required to help them to develop their own insight and understanding, to enable them to respond appropriately to the inner world of the foster child or young person.

The discussion explored the understanding of attachment and the meaning of integration, transference and countertransference, and therapeutic practice. These concepts were clarified and examples given by both Tom and Ann of the children and young people that they had fostered. They were able to reflect on the practical effects and impact on the children, though they were not always clear on the terminology or reasons behind the concepts.

The following shows part of the discussion and examples given:

> Even if the foster child is aged 8 years or above, it could be that in their internal world of emotions and capacity to function, they are still functioning at the level of an infant. It is then helpful for child if the foster parent can also provide for the lost and isolated small child inside them. In order for attachment to take place, the child will need to become absolutely dependent on the foster parent, and to feel that they are held in the mind of the foster parent. In time the child will begin to value the experience they have with the foster parent and start to move towards a meaningful attachment relationship. It is crucial for a traumatised child to feel held in the mind of the foster carer if they are to value and make positive use of their placement.

The difference in fostering an unintegrated compared to an integrated child or young person was discussed. Children who have been emotionally traumatised in their early life because they were not able to emotionally bond positively with their parents are left feeling emotionally isolated. Consequently, in their developing years their sense of self is not able to strengthen, and they become consumed with feelings which they are unable to communicate; and volatile emotions of panic and rage, which are very different from depressive emotions of sadness and anger. They feel emotionally and physically persecuted by the outside world, and inevitably respond by attacking others in return.

In contrast, a more integrated child is able to communicate and perhaps did not experience early trauma to the same degree as unintegrated children did, and as a consequence is able to maintain a balance between their internal world and the external world. Importantly, they are more able to express ambivalence, communicate their emotions to others, and relate to others in a group setting. They are also more able to learn from their experiences and maintain attachments and friendships.

Understanding the importance of transference and countertransference was of particular interest to Tom and Ann and one that mirrored their experiences.

Transference is the process by which the child or young person transfers onto the foster parent feelings and ideas, which belong to previous (often traumatic) experience they have endured in the past. If, for example, the child had experienced abuse and hostility from their previous carers, and the current foster parent become reactive to their behaviour, they could experience them as becoming as attacking and they may attack back. It is important that the foster parent has some insight into **who** the child is trying to recreate and not allow themselves to become the attacking parent, but rather to respond to the emotional pain and fear that the child may be feeling and expressing.

Countertransference denotes feelings and ideas which emerge within the foster parent themselves in response to the child's transference towards the foster parent. It is important that the foster parent has the opportunity and space to understand what the child or young person's behaviour brings up for them and to reflect on what it means for them. The hurt and pain of the child could bring out painful memories the foster parent holds about their own experiences, and it is important that they have the opportunity to reflect on these.

The importance of communication was clearly understood by both foster parents, and reinforced by Tom who stated,

> Communication is key to our house and our approach to fostering talking openly, not being judgemental and helping them to work through any negative behaviours. This isn't always a quick fix so acceptance is also very important.

All children and young people can communicate to varying degrees, but some are so overwhelmed with the pain and anxiety that they simply do not have the words to express themselves and say how they feel. There are, however, other ways through which the child can communicate, but if these are not understood by the foster parents, the child can easily break down and their unbearable feelings will be acted out destructively or self-destructively. There are three ways children and young people can communicate: verbal, non-verbal, and symbolic.

Non-verbal communication: A child whose early development has been halted because of early traumas and emotional abandonment has not been able to develop the words to express themselves. It is important that those responsible for their care can recognise parts of their difficult behaviour as a way of expressing their frustrations and upsets about reality. It is important that they have the help to respond to some of their unbearable expressions until words can start to express their emotions.

Symbolic communication: It can be a way of communication for traumatised children in infancy to make contact with reality. This can occur through play, the use of imagination, creating stories, dance, and drama. It can be a therapeutic road through for children and young people who are not yet able to use words to express themselves. It can be a good starting point for them and once recognised by foster parents, a way for the foster parent of making appropriate responses to them enabling them to connect and communicate with the child. I gave an anonymous example, based on Jess, where her dance and drama activity helped her to communicate more about her own inner struggles than she was able to articulate verbally at this point in time. In explaining the development from symbolic to verbal communication, I reflected that as she starts to strengthen emotionally, she will gain the confidence to communicate more through the use of words.

Verbal communication: A child or young person who is emotionally integrated and has a developing sense of self has the capacity to bring thinking and feelings together through words. At this point, a child who can communicate verbally is ready to use child psychotherapy to help them to reach the next stage of understanding more about their emotional life.

I met with Jess and the team who were responsible for her six months after I had originally spent time with her. The overall view was that she was now more settled, was functioning continually, and was more positive about her future than when I first met her. Generally, they informed me that she had evolved to a position where her emotional development was focused on how she felt about herself and, importantly, that she could communicate with them when she was feeling overwhelmed with emotions. Jess told me that she did feel much safer in the home than when I first met her, but that there were times when she did not know what do to with herself and she felt in a state of turmoil when she needed help to protect herself.

Although Jess continues to need some help to understand her strengths and weaknesses in her day-to-day living, she presented herself to me as a 'real self' who felt vulnerable at times, rather than the very fragmented child she was when I first met her. This illustrates how the concepts underpinning well-formulated therapeutic practice can be used to strengthen the emotional development and sense of self of a traumatised child.

Conclusion

This chapter has examined the complexities children and young people bring with them when they are being placed into a new family setting which offers them a very different experience than that of their original family environment. Although they desperately want a family who can offer them nurture and a sense of belonging as Jess outlined to me, they do not have the emotional resources to be able to value it. Often, they seek to destroy their placement, because internally they often do not feel worthy of any good experiences from a family setting. Long-term fostering is an important and valuable task for foster parents. However, there are a number of emotionally difficult ups and downs they have to go through before the child or young person can start to make a secure attachment relationship with the foster parents.

Although much has been written about meeting the emotional needs of traumatised children in a family setting, the key to achieving positive long-term outcomes for them is by helping them to believe and value that they now have a family where they feel they truly belong. It is within this family setting that they can find a new start in life for their future development with a sense of self which feels truly valued. The task for the foster parent is to provide good primary experiences for traumatised children and young children in their care, thus enabling them to reach the secondary stage of their maturational development positively and with a stronger sense of self.

It is crucial that residential workers who are preparing children and young people for foster placements have the appropriate training and professional support that will introduce them to the key elements of therapeutic concepts which will develop their capacity to respond to some of the more complex behaviour patterns of the young people for whom they are responsible. Importantly, this training can be used to support foster parents to develop their own insight, understanding, and responses in managing the painful and difficult behaviour of the foster children in their care who are overwhelmed with the emotions that result from the traumatic experiences they have endured.

Chapter 6

Providing an emotionally secure base for children and young people in secure children's homes and youth justice settings

The book has examined how the emotional turmoil for children and young people who have experienced intense traumatic experiences during the early stages of their life affects their capacity to manage the stresses and challenges of external reality as they grow up. The impact of these traumatic experiences is arrested emotional development. It has been acknowledged that appropriate Needs Led Assessment and Treatment Plan programmes can provide workers with some insight and understanding which can be used to help those they are responsible for to reach a more solid sense of self from which they feel they can function. Importantly, this offers the children and young people the capacity to manage their lived reality, not only during their current placement, but also with the ability to maintain it later when they have moved on to live in different and increasingly challenging environments.

This chapter explores whether the confinement of young people placed either in a secure children's home (SCH) or in youth justice settings actually addresses the emotional needs of children or young people who may be classified as 'frozen' or 'fragmented' displaying disorganised attachment and avoidant enmeshed attachment. It is important to understand the meaning of these two terms in order to recognise the impact on the child's sense of self, their behaviour, and the way that they interact with the outside world. These elements lie at the root of what brings the child or young person into secure children's homes (SCHs) and incarceration in young offending institutions (YOIs). The difference in terms of where the child or young person is placed depends on the severity of behaviour and whether they come before the family court system or the criminal justice system. Where a child or young person's behaviour is judged as being a risk to themselves or they are at risk of running away, the family court can issue an order for the young person to be placed in a secure children's home for a designated period of time. In contrast, a child or young person whose actions bring them before a criminal justice system court for judgement will be given a custodial sentence in a young offenders' institution.

The concept of an emotionally 'frozen' child as described in Chapter 2 relates to a child whose experience of infantile abuse and trauma commencing in the first few months of life and extending into childhood has been so extreme that it interrupts their emotional development. Instead of internalising a sense of trust and

DOI: 10.4324/9781003132882-9

connection with their primary carer, the child experiences and internalises feelings of annihilation and being attacked by others, and perceives the world as unpredictable, inconsistent, and one over which they have no control.

Over my many years of work with children and young people, I have often come across a number who have been placed in secure units and youth justice settings because of their anti-social behaviour, and on assessing them, I have found that they have been functioning at the level of a frozen child. As a reaction to the difficulty of managing the pressures of external reality which they find unbearable to think about, or manage, they have built up what has been described a 'false self' (Winnicott, 1969). The false self is confusing for carers and adults working with frozen children who find that they are faced with a dichotomy. The young person can present as charming and compliant, but as soon as they feel threatened, they can act out their panic and rage through violent and destructive behaviour by attacking others. The difficulty is that if residential settings develop a culture and practice which do not have an understanding of the impact of early trauma upon the child's internal world of thinking, and their inability to accept personal responsibility for their behaviour, the child's behaviour will continue to escalate. This results in placements continuing to break down and their youth offending behaviour progressing.

In contrast, a 'fragmented' child is described as a child or young person who had the opportunity to experience short periods of 'good enough care' as an infant and small child, which enabled them to flourish because they felt emotionally contained by their carer. However, this was short-lived, and the 'good enough care' was then replaced by the opposite when the child felt abused and abandoned both emotionally and physically by their carer. The result was that the child's own sense of self became fragmented, and their capacity to function and manage the challenges of external reality floundered when under stress. This type of experience has a direct impact on the child's maturational development, resulting in the child experiencing emotional gaps that prevent them from functioning in their day-to-day living. The impact is profound and can lead the young person to become locked away and ceasing to function. If fragmented children and young people are to manage the stresses of external reality, they inevitably require a great deal of support from those responsible for them in their placements. The young person anticipates failure when under stress and needs a great deal of support to survive the unbearable sense of loss and fears of abandonment that they experience. Although there are times when they can function well when they are faced with stress factors, without good support from their carer, they can fall into feelings of despair and depression, becoming self-destructive and self-harming when their self-esteem disintegrates. My experience is that secure children's homes and youth offending institutions comprise predominantly of frozen and fragmented children and young people.

An adolescent girl who had been assessed as a fragmented child when placed in a youth offending institution once said to me 'Either I want to dance all night and put my pretty dresses on, feeling lovely and having some fun, or, I want to hide in a dark hole where I feel that I can never escape from'. She was trying to explain to me how her life swung from one extreme to another in a way that was out of her control, and how she was not able to manage the stress of reality factors in her life. She needed a great deal of help and support from her carers to realise that she could manage boundaries without feeling that others were trying to attack her. She eventually came to the realisation that her level of self-esteem was so low that the slightest stress in her life could prevent her from functioning; such was the depth of her own underlying sense of worthlessness and hopelessness.

Explaining the relationship between the background and functioning of trauma-tised children and young people reveals the enormity of a task faced by workers to be able to use this understanding therapeutically to make a difference to the lives of these young people. It is important to ask, how can workers be helped to achieve the depth of insight and understanding needed to work therapeutically with these young people especially when they are placed in secure children's homes and youth treatment centres? The complex histories and needs of this vulnerable group of young people question whether current solutions of incarceration actually work. Does incarceration offer a physical and emotional environment that engen-ders a sense of personal development and responsibility? Or, does it, in contrast, exacerbate existing anti-social behaviours and mental health issues and potentially encourage what has been described in Chapter 5 as a delinquent merger (enmeshed attachment) where the personal boundaries in a relationship between two or more young people are permeable and unclear? Workers are faced with young people whose complex and chaotic lives place both themselves, and others physically and emotionally, at risk. The task faced by those responsible for young people whether in secure units or youth justice settings is difficult and often comes at a heavy cost to themselves. Workers may find themselves overwhelmed by the task they face and may find it difficult to make a positive impact on the lives of these young peo-ple. However, a key question needs to be addressed, namely:

Is the fundamental purpose of these institutions one of 'protecting society', or, do they acknowledge a responsibility to 're-educate' and work therapeutically to care for the mental health of these young people, and work towards countering the escalation of behaviours that may lead from a secure children's home place-ment, to custody in a young offenders' institution, and from a young offenders' institution to recidivism and adult prison?

Young people between the ages of 10 and 17 whose behaviour poses a risk to them-selves, to others, or are at risk of running away can be subject to a Section 25 of the 1989 Children's Act family court secure order for placement in a secure children's home. In an emergency, a young person may be detained for three days without a court order, but one must be applied for placement of a child for a longer period of up to a year. In contrast, young people of a similar age who have broken the law can be held in custody in a young offenders' institution. A key concern is whether the secure children's home is able to address the complexity of the young person's needs during the time they are being held, to enable them to return to fostering or residential care successfully, rather than their behaviour escalating to the point where they break the law and are sentenced to a young offenders' institution.

Other than the degree of escalation, the background of young people who are subject to custody in a secure children's home and a young offenders' institution is similar. Both are characterised by early experiences of trauma, abuse, and neglect, difficulties settling, and a number of placements, mostly in residential rather than family placement, and often a recent placement move within the last year (Hart and LaValle, 2016:19). For most children who are being considered for a secure placement, the origins of their risky behaviour lies in early childhood experiences, such as abuse, neglect, parental rejection, or loss, but they were late entrants to the care system. This raises questions about whether more could have been done, both prior to their becoming looked after and in previous placements, to prevent their distress from escalating to the point where they needed to be 'held' in order to keep them safe (Hart and LaValle, 2016:10).

Taylor (2016:2) in his review of the youth justice system in England and Wales reported that among the children within the criminal justice system,:

> a large proportion have previously been in care (38% in Young Offender Institutions, 52% in Secure Training Centres), and more than a third have a diagnosed mental health disorder. Many of the children in the system come from some of the most dysfunctional and chaotic families where drug and alcohol misuse, physical and emotional abuse and offending is common.

The complexity of their backgrounds is again acknowledged by the Prison Reform Trust (2015:4), which noted that:

> Looked-after children are more likely to be exposed to the risk factors established in research and associated with the onset of youth offending rather than the general population of children. Risk factors for youth crime, and the factors leading to reception into care are similar. Risk (and protective) factors for young people who offend are categorised across four domains: the family; school; community; and those which are individual, personal, and related to peer group experiences. The majority of children in care are from backgrounds of deprivation, poor parenting, abuse and neglect – factors that together create risk for a range of emotional, social and behavioural difficulties, including anti-social and offending behaviour.

Whilst a secure placement was usually seen as effective in stabilising children and keeping them safe, subsequent outcomes were reported as being 'mixed' and there were different opinions as to whether SCHs can realistically be expected to address the underlying causes of the children's behaviour. There appears to be a particular gap in services for children with attachment, conduct, emerging personality, or post-traumatic stress disorders, with these children falling between social care and health provision (Hart and LaValle, 2016:10).

A critical element of confinement relates to the experiences of the young person once in a young offenders' institution, and whether the routines, support and provision available, are sufficiently 'child-focused'. The use of, and effectiveness of, for example, Separation orders (under Rule 49), which although time-limited, specifies that separation is used:

> where it appears desirable, for the maintenance of good order or discipline or in his own interests, that an inmate should not associate with other inmates, either generally or for particular purposes, the governor may arrange for the inmate's removal from association accordingly.

The isolation of young people who are at risk to others or themselves, specifically in the case of frozen or fragmented children, is of concern under the conditions for separation, detailed above, and needs to be considered. Rather than being seen as 'punishment' that did not address escalations of behaviour, the 2020 Separation Taskforce listed 13 recommendations, including:

RECOMMENDATION 3: The purpose of separation should be defined and support a change in culture so that it is seen and experienced as a positive intervention.

RECOMMENDATION 13: The considerable role of health, education, and other services to support separated children within a multidisciplinary framework for integrated care should be clarified, so they have access to the regime and services they require. Governors and service provider partners need to work in a focused and fully integrated manner to enable children to have access to a fuller regime when they are separated.

Given the recommendations that have been made about providing the appropriate provision required to meet the needs of children and young people in need of secure children's homes or youth justice settings, the following questions need to be considered: how can workers develop a culture where children and young people who have become emotionally trapped because of early traumas and are not able to relate to others who are placed there, can thrive and develop? How is the difficult and at times aggressive behaviour of young people responded to by their workers? Do workers become controlling and reactive towards them, only to increase the children's destructive or self-destructive behaviour towards themselves and others? Ultimately, are workers able to respond with meaning to the young people, offering them ways of navigating their lives?

A way forward is to train workers to engage in the process of a therapeutic encounter with children and young people when they are placed in secure children's homes or youth justice settings. The purpose is to develop workers' understanding of the concepts of integrated and fragmented states of mind in children and young people and how these impact on the young person's behaviour. This will help the workers to live alongside the painful and unbearable emotions that the children and young people carry with them and support them to manage themselves in a more realistic way, however painful it is for them. The result is to show young people that they no longer have to act out their panic and rage, which can often lead to escalation of behaviour. In contrast, learning to share their own vulnerability, sadness, and despair with those who are responsible for them will help them to realise that there are people present who can listen, understand, and help to meet their emotional needs.

It is critical that appropriate training is identified which can give workers an understanding of the appropriate concepts which can help to deepen and strengthen their practice. Workers need to evaluate whether the young person's experience during their incarceration addresses the complexity of their needs since they cannot learn from their experiences because their sense of reality does not correspond to that of other people. If a severely traumatised child or young person has felt attacked and abused by those who were responsible for them in their early life, they respond by creating their own reality which does not fit in with external reality. Inevitably, stress can result in a breakdown of their behaviour when the child becomes overwhelmed with panic, rage, and unbearable anxiety which they are not able to think about, or even accept personal responsibility for their actions. An examination of the behaviours and the life histories of children and young people who are placed in secure children's homes or youth justice settings shows that they carry with them experiences of early trauma, neglect, privation, and abuse and can be classified as 'frozen' or 'fragmented' (disorganised attachment/ avoidant enmeshed attachment). Examination of these concepts and specialist training will provide insight into the behaviour and thinking of this group of young people and propose ways forward to challenge re-offending and recidivism and the likelihood of progression into youth offending institutions.

The important questions that must be asked here are: What are we looking for from the placement of children and young people in secure unit children's homes and youth justice settings? What do we call good outcomes? Currently, the degree of recidivism where young people repeat youth offending and returning to youth offending centres is high. It is critical that the culture of the home or treatment centre does not collude in allowing young people who are characterised as having what Winnicott (1963) described as a 'false self', to be held without appropriate therapeutic treatment and support. This 'false self' means that the young person has the capacity to comply with the rules of the culture at a superficial level, but without any fundamental change and so as soon as they leave the setting, they continue to repeat the anti-social tendency because nothing has changed. What needs to be examined is the long-term view of those young people after their placement has come to an end to ascertain whether the intervention has been successful.

In order to gain a broader sense of perspective, it is important to look at earlier attempts to address the complex needs of young people whose experiences of trauma were compounded by multiple placements in residential children's homes or foster placements and to identify what can be learnt from exemplars of this early provision. During 1970–1980, I worked in the Cotswold Community, which at the time was similar to a youth justice setting today but radically changing its approach to how they work with young offenders by adopting a more therapeutic approach. It created a culture that was truly focused on the importance of under-standing and meeting the young person's emotional needs, in an environment that was able to provide the appropriate therapeutic provision for them. Although the Cotswold Community no longer exists, it is worth mentioning the impact that the community philosophy and practice had on both the young people and the workers themselves. The result of the changes the community leadership undertook in help-ing workers to be able to live alongside the panic, rage, and feelings of despair that the adolescents carried with them was put into practice. The therapeutic concepts they were learning were profound. It resulted in both the young people and the workers feeling and believing that they were part of a community that they wanted to be part of and who provided them with a secure base from which they could develop as individuals. It took ten years of sound therapeutic working practice to turn the community around. Recidivism where young people returned to prison or youth offending centres had lessened from 85% when it was an approved school, to 0.5% after the culture had become a secure base from which those placed there could develop their own sense of self in a more real and meaningful way.

These two examples offer important insight into the long-term impact of thera-peutic provision:

Alan reflected that although it had been 50 years since his placement at the Cotswool School (which today would be described as a secure children's home or youth justice setting), he had been drawn back to memories of the time he spent there and had nothing but fond memories of his stay. He said that he held nothing but respect for it. Although he had been through a number of difficult times in his life since leaving, he was now firmly safe and secure in his own personal and professional life. As he began to think about it again, tears came to his eyes. He continued to hold a clear and profound respect for the help he received during his time there.

John described his time at the community and school as giving him a firm foun-dation from which he was able to develop his life. He said that he learnt how to interact with others and behave in what he called 'a civilised manner' and not engage with conflict situations, but instead work with conflict resolution. He acknowledged that his time at the community had helped him to thrive and become the person he is today.

Of course, it is always inspiring to read about how good positive experiences in a residential placement helped the child or young person to become more emotionally positive about themselves, with the outcome being that they are able to internalise their experiences and use these to strengthen their relationship with external reality. However, we must also be aware that there will be some who did not have the same outcome experience as those described earlier. The question that must be asked again is: what is the provision today for children and young people who are placed into specialist secure unit or youth justice setting placements, and critically, whether it is 'fit for purpose'? Currently, conceptual thinking is very clear about the impact of early traumatic experiences on a young child and the impact it has on their ability to successfully integrate the challenges of the outside world becoming able to manage the reality factors they have to face. We must also question how do the concepts become placed into good practice, where the traumatised child or young person really feels that they are being held in the mind of the workers. It is not an easy task for workers to be able to live alongside some of the most unbearable and unthinkable emotions, which lie in the minds of those for whom they are responsible and where workers have the insight and experience to manage issues such as transference and countertransference successfully without personal risk and emotional burnout. The long-term success lies in young people developing a strengthened sense of self as a result of their experiences and relationships developed with other children or young people and the workers, during their secure placement.

However, recent reports of secure units do not appear to reflect conceptual change and concepts that reflect good practice such as being 'held in mind' or working towards strengthening a young person's sense of self and the development of healthy relationships.

The inspection report of one YOI (2021) highlighted a number of key concerns, which critically mirror the unaddressed chaos of the inner worlds of children and young incarcerated. These included:

1.36: The number of violent incidents was high. The response to this was invariably to keep children apart from each other, which had a negative impact on their regime and reinforced the violent behaviour. Staffing unavailability, lack of engagement and redeployment of specialist conflict resolution staff to support the regime compounded the problem (2021:13).

1.37: Too much poor behaviour went unchallenged by staff. This included banging of doors, the blocking of observation panels and shouting out of doors and windows. Expectations of behaviour were not enforced robustly and there was an inconsistent approach to ensuring that even the most basic of standards were met. There was a lack of immediate or longer-term rewards or incentives to reward good behaviour and make sure that children who engaged could consistently progress and attain long-term goals both within the prison – for example, with a more trusted status – or as they moved toward release (2021:13).

1.39: Extensive and offensive graffiti in cells, communal areas and exercise yards remained a significant problem and was emblematic of generally poor standards across the prison. During the inspection, children told us that graffiti was a 'normal' feature of the prison. Poor standards of cleanliness in cells and communal areas were not challenged effectively by staff and managers (2021:13).

3.36: We observed assaults and fights throughout the inspection, often erupting simply in response to name calling or because children on the units were from different sub-groups. Paradoxically, the act of reducing group sizes to reduce violence had created yet more division and conflict among the children. Of concern was the frequency of multiple perpetrator assaults, where two or more children would attack a lone child simultaneously.

Throughout the residential units, staff strictly controlled the unlocking of any cell door while children from a different sub-group were on the landing. This reflected a lack of staff confidence in managing individual children, and the widespread belief that children would attack each other at any opportunity.

(2021:25–26)

The extracts cited here suggest that nurturing and the opportunity to develop positive relationships appeared to be minimal, and were reinforced by the fact that time out of their cell was limited, restricted to a daily average of about four and half hours on weekdays and two hours at weekends (2021:14), and that young people ate most of their meals alone in their cell. They were only able to access a maximum of 12 hours of education per week, but for many, it was far less with poor attendance at education classes. Children did not undertake enough learning outside formal education lessons. They felt frustrated, justifiably, that they spent too much time in their cell without doing anything purposeful (2021:11). This is of additional concern given that each young person under the age of 18, given their background, should have an Education, Health and Care Plan (EHCP). The EHCP within the SEND code of practice (DfE and NHS, 2015) is a legally binding document outlining a child or young person's special educational, health, and social care needs and describes the extra support to be given and how their needs will be met. It not only applies to schools, local authorities, Child and Adolescent Mental Health Services (CAMHS) support, and NHS (2015:40) but importantly applies to youth offending teams and relevant youth custodial establishments (2015:13) comprising young offending institutions, secure training centres, secure children's homes, or secure colleges.

Given what has been discussed about frozen and fragmented children and young people, how does current provision such as that described here, which is focused on incarceration, help to reform their behaviour, develop their sense of self, and address the issue of potential recidivism?

To help me to understand the real-life experience of a young person whose early life led ultimately to incarceration, I met with Jay to discuss with him about the times he had spent in a youth offending institution and prisons.

He shared his experiences with me. Jay had been through a very troubled and traumatic early home life, which had left him with a sense of emotional isolation within himself. He said that he did not know who he really was or where he belonged, and this led him into becoming part of a gang culture who were involved with criminal and at times quite violent activities. Eventually, he was arrested and placed into a young offenders' institution and later served two prison sentences. Even in the middle of this, Jay hoped to receive some help for himself. He continued to feel completely lost in the prison environments, where he found that a number of the inmates were working towards forming gang cultures in their prison or young offenders' institutions. The only way to avoid being drawn into these new gangs, which he did not wish to be a part of, was to isolate himself remaining on his own for long periods of time.

Jay then told me about the ways in which groups of adolescents found ways of 'merging' with each other and creating sub-cultures and gangs whilst they continued to present themselves as being compliant to their workers or prison officers. In this way, the workers or officers would never be in touch with the complex dynamics, which were occurring in the group setting. It also meant that they could continue to develop sub-cultural activities within the group. Such anti-social group dynamics makes it very difficult for vulnerable children and young people to survive in these settings, and it was of little surprise that a number of them became suicidal and self-harming whilst they were placed there. It was inevitable that during his placements, Jay began to feel lost within himself as did many other young people, because the only options of managing unbearable feelings and thoughts which could not be communicated about to the workers or officers responsible for them, were either to join the gang culture or to become self-harming and suicidal.

To deal with his own feelings of self-isolation, Jay had the courage to join the youth council in the prison. This he felt was very helpful to him, because he wanted to feel that he was trying to help something to change in the prison system and a very useful way out of being thrown into the sub-cultural practices in the system. Rather than becoming lost in the pitfalls of the dynamics of the prison and youth offending institute, he wanted to look at what was going on in the prisons rather than becoming a part of it. He also believed that life was at times so unbearable, difficult, and painful for some of the prisoners and young people that they created their own reality which could become destructive or self-destructive quite often, and not what was expected by them during the time they spent in their incarceration. Jay believed that becoming a member of the youth council was a way forward for him to try to repair some of the difficult circumstances in which he and other young people found themselves. As part of the youth council, he felt he had a powerful 'voice' where, as one of them, he could speak to inmates, listen to what they had to say, and raise issues for change on their behalf, before the prison panel.

Jay told me that eventually when he left prison, he engaged with a therapist who was able to help him understand and make sense of his experiences and think more about himself.

After spending some time with Jay, I asked him what he had learnt from his experiences in the three placements he went through, and what he felt could be learnt to make them better for the young offenders who were placed there.

He suggested that it was important to identify:

- How life in the young offender and prison settings can change to work more positively for offenders.
- The key issues in the establishments that need working on.
- What needs to be done for workers and officers to help them understand more about meeting the emotional needs of those they are responsible for, and to communicate with them more positively and thoughtfully.

To respond to Jay appropriately, I have set out my own thoughts to offer guidance about the need for change in young offender and prison settings.

1 If young offender training centres and prisons are to understand and provide for meeting both the emotional and realistic needs of young offenders, we need to discuss how the provision offered to them can recognise and facilitate fundamental requirements to support their day-to-day living. To be successful, we need to define and consider the emotional, social, and physical needs of these young people. It is crucial that their time in a youth treatment centre or prison is internalised and taken in by them as an experience resulting in them feeling and believing that they matter as an individual in their own right during their stay. When they have completed their stay, they should have acquired a stronger sense of self within themselves, and with continued support, can find managing the challenges of the external world and reality factors more manageable than they had originally. From my experience of the complexities of the culture of youth offending centres, this is undoubtedly a great challenge for providers, but crucial if both the primary and secondary tasks of YOIs and prisons are to be successful.

2 It is important that the primary and secondary needs of young offenders can be recognised and assessed. Importantly, as Gooch (2019:81) observes, 'juvenile prisoners, by virtue of the Children's Act 1989, are still children but are held within a very "adult prison environment where they are defined first and foremost as a prisoner"', a concern raised originally by Taylor (2016) in his review of the juvenile justice system. One of the main key issues that needs to be addressed by workers when planning to meet the needs of young people who have offended is to be able to acknowledge the level of their emotional development. It is important to recognise that many of these adolescents or young people placed in secure children's homes, youth training centres, or prisons carry the legacy of early trauma. This trauma has a detrimental impact on their emotional development which remains stuck at the level of a small child even though they are physically mature. It is crucial that workers are trained to recognise some of their difficult behaviour as a sign of the panic, rage, and despair which they at times act out aggressively or self-destructively and belong to a period of their earlier life when they were overwhelmed with unbearable and unthinkable anxieties. The majority of children and young people whether in secure unit children's homes, YOIs, and prisons have been through a breakdown of their placements in residential care fostering and adoption placements. With insight and understanding, workers will be able to respond rather than react to their behaviour and, in so doing, offer a positive way forward.

3 What can be offered to workers and prison officers if they are to understand more about the complex behaviour of young offenders and be able to respond accordingly to their needs? Specialist training is essential to help them understand more about the internal world of children and young people who have been

traumatised and re-traumatised by both their early experiences and experiences whilst growing up, and consequently have little or no positive belief in themselves and external reality. Four important aspects of child and adolescent development are advised:

- Transference and countertransference in work with traumatised children and young people.
- Understanding the concept of the frozen child.
- Ego-support and ego-provision in a therapeutic environment.
- Communication: verbal, non-verbal, and symbolic.

It is not only training courses they require but also how to apply their learning and transform it into meaningful therapeutic practice, one that enables young people to make sense of experiences and their lives. Sadie *et al.* (2022:5) reflect that:

> We often notice that children in custody lack a coherent narrative of their life experiences, but beyond this, it is clear that incarceration – particularly when it is long term, or indeterminate, poses an overwhelming oncological threat. "Who am I. if this is happening, who can I be now? What happens to my relationships my hopes and plan?

This chapter has explored the complexities of recreating a positive therapeutic culture which can identify and reach out, address, and meet the emotional needs of young people in secure children's homes and young offender institutions. There is considerable evidence to suggest that those placed there have been engaged in destructive sub-cultural activities, which carry their own norms, culture, ethnicity, sexuality, and values, prior to their incarceration, and which they inevitably bring with them to their new placement. Hilder *et al.* (2021) gathered together the life histories of 81 prolific robbery offenders with an emphasis on diverse childhood experiences including victimisation by parents or other adults. They reported that of the 81 in their study, 80% had been victims of crime and violence themselves. Given patterns of behaviour and experiences such as these, the only positive way to prevent sub-cultural groups forming in settings where youth offenders are concentrated is for the placement environment to have a countering culture, which is focused on identifying and facilitating the meeting of the emotional needs of the young people incarcerated.

It is important to accept that the culture in which we are raised plays a critical role in shaping who we are and what we perceive as normal or odd about our lives. Therefore, it is crucial that secure children's homes and young offender institutions develop a culture that workers and young people are engaged with, one that offers positive alternatives.

The professional workers that I have spoken to are totally committed to developing a stronger therapeutic practice, and it appears that there is a general commitment to bringing in a stronger therapeutic approach to the emotional containment of young offenders. However, it is recognised that it is a long hard struggle to bring the theory and practice together and create a positive therapeutic approach to their work with severely emotionally damaged children and young offenders. A change in culture is required, one that acknowledges how hard it is to help workers to deal with their own anxieties and uncertainties about the work with children and young offenders who themselves are overwhelmed with panic, rage, and unbearable anxieties and who can act out their emotions destructively or self-destructively.

Currently, little thought has been given to implementing practice, which focuses on the emotional needs of these young people, but finding the starting point is fundamental to the difficult and complex work required by those who are committed to making it work. My earlier description of the Cotswold Community many years ago shows that this approach does work and has a long-term impact. I can only assure the workers and practitioners in the field that it is worth the struggle and hard work for the long-term outcomes of the work to be successful. Where those working in these complex settings are committed to developing good practice at all levels for those working there, in time, the culture will grow and positive change will happen.

Chapter 7

Finding their way

Helping and supporting unaccompanied refugee and asylum-seeking children and young people to settle

NCHR, UNICEF, and IOM (2019) reported that at the end of 2019, of the 32,200 children who came into Europe, 9,000 were unaccompanied asylum-seeking children under the age of 18 years of whom 3,550 came to the UK. These young unaccompanied refugees and asylum seekers are faced with painful and difficult traumas that they have to endure and learn to manage in their quest for establishing a new life for themselves. This is particularly so when they finally settle in a new country where the cultural, political, and psychological factors are quite different realities from their own. Although their journey to safety is driven by hope, the physical and emotional pain experienced by these children can be quite overwhelming, particularly where it is accompanied by persecution, intimidation, and violence. As unaccompanied minors, they may experience not only the unimaginable loss of family, friends, and their community, but also the loss of their home language and the learning of a new language that they have to manage. Once having arrived in this country, without the safety-net of their family and community, they can find themselves being subjected to poverty, loneliness, and discrimination in addition to experiencing a loss of self-esteem, status, and identity. It is also important to acknowledge how the crossing of continents and countries can leave them vulnerable, in danger, and at risk of being exploited either into slave labour or being trafficked. Critically, their vulnerability can be compounded, leaving their capacity for resilience broken.

Their resilience is further compromised where they carry family histories of violence, cruelty, and sexual violation and have not experienced good enough early experiences of their own to draw on (Trowell, 2002:102). Children and young people who experienced trauma and abuse in their family environments can view their current experiences of being a refugee as reflecting the same reality of having to survive in a hostile environment, as that originally experienced in their early life. Their response and defence will be either attacking others destructively, or engaging in self-destructive behaviour towards themselves. This places them at great risk, because their insecurity is rooted in the fact that they did not feel securely held in the mind of their primary carer causing them to feel abused and emotionally abandoned. As a consequence, they are unable to share the world with others

DOI: 10.4324/9781003132882-10

or manage the challenges of external reality which can be painful for them at times. Their sense of self is so fragile that they are unable to emotionally integrate their experiences in their new country nor manage the current realities they are facing. Life can become very overwhelming for them and can lead to them breaking down mentally or physically.

In contrast, children who show resilience and have the capacity to cope with the trauma of migration are ones who have had early positive nurturing experiences of love and emotional security from their families. It is this group, as young people, who will have the ability and confidence to build friendships and find a place for themselves in a supportive community. Achieving a sense of belonging, including having positive ethnic identities, valuing their personal identity, having a positive outlook (Pieloch et al., 2016:387), and having the capacity for resilience, is key to the child's ability to survive and thrive in a new environment and culture. The quality of their primary relationship determines the child's level of emotional integration (being able to bring feelings and thinking together). This enables them to hold onto feelings of trust and safety, having internalised a secure base because of the emotional richness and strength they experienced from their primary attachment and relationship with their carer.

The migration experience, nevertheless, makes mental health one of the key issues that must be addressed to support the successful integration of migrant children and young people into their host communities. This is especially true of refugee children who have a higher prevalence of both exposure to traumatic events and higher levels of mental health symptoms such as post-traumatic stress disorders (PTSD) and depression compared to the general population (Abdi, 2018:337).

The DFE guidance (2017:3) given to local authorities for the care of vulnerable unaccompanied migrant children and child victims who have been trafficked and are at risk of modern slavery is that they have a duty to protect and support them through the local authority care system. In addition to the risk they face, the complexity of their needs and trauma experienced requires that local authority support must begin as soon as the child is referred to the local authority, or is found in their area.

The child or young person's initial experiences when arriving in their new country are that of being placed in an Immigration Removal Centre before finding the necessary help and emotional support they require if they are to develop a solid base for themselves from which they can start to build and strengthen their new lives. Their experience may be complicated by the need for a formal age assessment especially where the child does not have personal documentation with them. Although the Home Office guidance asserts that detention and removal are essential to ensure effective immigration control, it also pledges that decisions to detain them are never taken lightly, and states that detainees must be treated with dignity and detention must be used sparingly (Crawley and Lester, 2005). Refugee and asylum-seeking children should have the chance to feel safe and happy and to have a chance for a positive and successful life in their new country, regardless of their parent's immigration status.

Whatever the practical elements of their new status, it must be acknowledged that all of the children and young people who arrive in their new country also carry with themselves their own internal world of feelings, thoughts, and ideas from having both positive and painful experiences in their life so far. They carry with them memories of what led to them leaving their home, country, and culture. The difficulty for them is that the external realities they have to face up to and manage can be extremely difficult and painful, and they are inevitably drawn back to the feelings that originate with experiences of earlier trauma. They will need to learn a new language and settle into a foster home or residential care. If older, they must find accommodation, and manage school or learning in further education and forming new friendships, whilst also tackling the challenges and powerlessness of the bureaucratic procedures, which they may have to navigate themselves. Although the current support system may provide them with a great amount of the support and care dealing with all the areas they have to face, they may still feel a sense of personal isolation and loneliness. For some, this can become unbearable and at times turn into a case of depressive survival. The role played by workers in helping young people to break out of this cycle of despair is critical. They offer a sense of community and a place where young people can talk openly about their experiences to people that they trust.

Working with refugee and unaccompanied children and young people is a complex process and painful for workers who are required to engage meaningfully with them whilst maintaining their own personal and professional barriers to avoid engaging in transference and countertransference, and ultimately burnout. A common thread throughout this book has been to highlight the importance for workers to develop a deeper understanding about the internal world of traumatised children and young people. In doing so, they will help these young people to balance the need to meet the expectations of the external reality in their lives, whilst also managing their own internal anxieties and fears, uncertainties, and insecurities.

My time spent with the three specialist refugee charity organisations who are pre-occupied with understanding and meeting the practical and emotional needs of refugee and asylum-seeking children and young people was invaluable. The enormity and complexity of their task in hand left me deeply thoughtful and reflective. The level of pre-occupation the teams have on understanding and responding to meeting the needs of all their clients is extensive. The young people's requirement for intervention is high because of the turbulent feelings they bring with them.

What then is the primary task of the organisations who work with refugee and asylum-seeking unaccompanied children and young people? What is the quality of therapeutic intervention? The following part of this chapter will explore how three specialist centres are developing their insight and understanding as to how they can reach out to and meet both the practical and emotional needs of these children and young people. They recognise that children on the move face many safety risks and concerns, from being separated from their families to the risk of sexual abuse and violence along dangerous travel routes.

The primary task articulated by the first specialist charity organisation that I met with was to:

- Empower each young person by building their resilience and the reconciliation of their trauma. To encourage and facilitate independence, self-reliance, and integration into local communities and UK society as a whole.
- Offer a comprehensive trauma-informed legal network to support individual asylum claims. This ensures that each young person's best interests and future choices are upheld and protected.
- Encourage relationship building and the bridging of cultural barriers. Our diverse and experienced staff team is on duty 24/7 and works to place young people into local schools as soon as possible whilst exploring the participation in academic and vocational opportunities and local community initiatives.

These are very well-founded and sincere statements, and undoubtedly, some young people for whom professional workers are responsible will experience success and achieve a sense of feeling valued by others. This can result in a better ability to function successfully in their new life. However, the following questions must be asked:

What about those young people who do not have access to specialist charities which provide therapeutic treatment and support for refugee and asylum-seeking children and young people?

How will these young people, without appropriate therapeutic intervention, be able to gain a stronger sense of self, from which they can move forward positively to the next stage of their lives in the new environment they live in?

Without the help of specialist charities engaged in therapeutic work, these young people cannot move forward psychologically, socially, or culturally, without breaking down or becoming destructive towards others, or self-destructive towards themselves. The knowledge required by the workers to engage with, and support young asylum seekers to turn their lives around, cannot be underestimated.

The level of emotional integration the child has reached determines their ability to manage and adapt to the culture of their new country as they learn to accept and live within a new set of rules. Central to the child's level of emotional development is the quality of their early primary relationship where thinking about their emotions can be worked through in a loving family environment. The child is able to internalise feelings of trust and safety, and although they will suffer a tragic sense of loss from having left their country and family environment, which felt secure and meaningful for them, they will have the capacity to draw strength from this. Although they will require a great amount of support and help to manage their depressive anxieties, in time they will be able to re-establish themselves in their current environment, finding a new starting point for the next stage of their lives.

Experience shows that with appropriate therapeutic treatment and support from those responsible for them in their new country, young people who have had early positive and caring family relationships can develop the capacity to work through their fears and anxieties, whereas those who remain deeply emotionally fragmented will find their capacity to function in their new environment very difficult and at times impossible to manage.

The level of emotional integration the child has reached determines their ability to manage and adapt to the culture in their new country as they learn to accept and live within a new set of rules. Central to the child's level of emotional integration is the quality of their early primary relationship. In a loving, supportive family environment, the child is able to internalise feelings and thoughts of trust and safety, and although they may suffer a tragic sense of loss of their previous life, they will have the capacity to draw strength from this. They may require a great amount of support and help to manage their depressive anxieties, but in time will be able to re-establish themselves in their current environment, finding a new starting point for the next stage of their lives.

However, a child who did not experience an internalised secure base from which they could function because of early experiences of neglect, trauma, and emotional abandonment, later coupled with exposure to violence, cruelty, and experience of war, is particularly vulnerable. Their inner world is ultimately driven by feelings of fury, sadness, and rage. Their emotions have become extreme and unbearable, and they are unable to think about or control them. At this point, the child over-identifies with the external reality of war and chaos, seeing them as reflections of their own inner world of overwhelming emotions and emotional abandonment by their carers. Their perception is that there is an all-consuming war between themselves and others, and their lack of emotional resources makes it very difficult for them to achieve age-related maturational development even in the safety of their new country. Understanding how to respond therapeutically to these young people who although overwhelmed by unbearable and painful feelings may present as charming and self-contained on the surface, but subject to breakdown under the slightest stress, is essential. It enables the worker to connect, to break through barriers and understand the symbolism and patterns of behaviours, and to begin the process where the young person is ready to see themselves and their future in a different way.

The second specialist charity that I met with described creating a planned therapeutic environment for these young people. They provided access to six levels of intervention, which was vital in enabling them to move towards the next stage of their transitional development. These comprised the following:

- Individual psychotherapy.
- Group psychotherapy.
- Access to case work and social work to help accessing housing benefits, work and education, and health care.
- Support through the prolonged asylum system.

- Attendance at community meetings and events and participation in their governance.
- A variety of arts and sports-based small therapeutic groups, including art and music and filmmaking, kayaking, climbing, and horse riding.

It was also recognised by the team that all the young asylum seekers attending their centre presented significant mental health, and developmental and psychosomatic symptoms after their experiences of extreme acts of organised and interpersonal violence. However, the team were able to show that they were able to provide an environment which met the emotional needs of the young people and make a real difference to their lives, even though this would need to continue for an extended period for it to have a long-term effect.

They were very clear about the outcomes that they sought for the young people that they worked with:

- To achieve a sense of belonging. Having a relationship with at least one adult who is emotionally in touch with them and who they feel held in mind by.
- Being able to discuss their difficulties at their level of understanding.
- Being able to learn to share difficulties and find solutions in discussions with others.
- Being able to shift from being stuck in various areas of their thinking and to be able to imagine and engage in new ways of being.
- After feeling a part of the community, they were living with, that they could eventually find a place of belonging in their community of exile and participation in community, life work, and relationships.

The following reflections from young asylum seekers at the Baobab Centre (Ellison, 2022) capture the fears, anxieties, and hopes they experienced whilst attempting to integrate themselves into their new lives and becoming able to function positively when they are placed into an entirely different culture from the ones they have lost.

> Even when I feel hopeless there is something inside me that will not give up. I don't know what it is, But I know it is there.
>
> I told myself you're not in Afghanistan now. There is no threat or bombs, it's safe, different governments, different rules.
>
> Empty your head, do your best each day, and learn new things.
>
> When I arrived, it felt like a different world. I missed my family and friends and worried about them. But slowly I have learned many things, like how to cope with my loneliness.
>
> Growing up I never belonged anywhere so I'm still not 100% here. I still fear what could happen. Confidence comes slowly.

These reflections convey some of the profound feelings of relief, fear, and uncertainty these young asylum seekers carry with them, all of which influence their emotional growth. However, what is clear is that with the appropriate support to emotionally and practically facilitate their needs, their experience of living in a new environment can provide a positive way forward, in spite of the extent of the trauma they carry with them.

To gain a deeper understanding of what it was like for young people who were trying to integrate themselves into a new community, culture and country, and the emotional struggles they experienced and dealt with in their search for a new beginning, I met with Hamid.

Hamid had been in England for two years after spending several years in a variety of countries having to flee on his own because of the war between different factions and cultures, and in which he saw numerous friends and family members killed. Hamid was in his early teens when he realised that he would have to leave his home country if he were to survive, and find a new life for himself from which he could develop. For Hamid, to make the decision was brave and courageous but it was not easy. He spent the following seven years in several different countries in Middle East, then Europe. He did any work to survive and in some countries was able to function and make friends. In other countries, he was tortured and spent time in harsh prisons where he experienced cruelty and violence. In spite of the traumatic times that he went through on his journey, Hamid never gave up on his determination to find a new home setting for himself, where he could eventually find a sense of belonging to the culture and become a part of the community. In 2020, he was able to come to the UK and start to find that new beginning for himself. Although the strength of Hamid's determination and resilience saw him through in spite of all that he suffered, there were still a number of critical factors that he had to deal with and manage on his own. Internally, he had to deal with feelings of loss and of being alone; also, he had to deal with the external reality and the barriers of the systems that he had to struggle through. These included the following:

- Receiving recognition as a refugee rather than a non-asylum seeker.
- Learning a new language.
- Finding accommodation for himself because he was over the age to be taken into the care system.
- Adapting to the new and different culture he was now living in and staying within their rules and regulations. This was difficult for him, and he had to think deeply about managing this, particularly after he had spent time in many different countries with different rules, customs, and behaviours.

In time, through his own resilience and determination to create a new life for himself, Hamid did manage to achieve success in all of these. Critically, he was also supported deeply and meaningfully by a refugee charity which he has continued to use, becoming a part of their community. Hamid has dealt with finding a starting point in his new life by becoming a part of a choir of refugees which helps him to feel a sense of belonging to a family, and importantly, he has also won a scholarship to start a degree at university.

However, in spite of the huge resilience and determination that Hamid has shown and that led him to achieve and establish himself in the UK, he was still left with recurring fears and anxieties that he has had to manage daily. As Hamid became more settled in his new home country, he started to dream more, with many of his past memories emerging. Some were good dreams about his early life with his family when he was a three-year-old playing with his siblings and family. Yet at times, his dreams could turn into nightmares, when memories of the struggles he had trying to escape from the unbearable traumas which he had to confront when he was left fighting for his life emotionally and physically. The most painful situation for him was having to live with past memories which continue to bombard him in spite of the way in which he has worked towards establishing a new life for himself.

I found Hamid's history moving and most inspirational to hear about. Although he now genuinely feels that he has found a new family environment and a sense of belonging to people who care for him, he does yet not feel completely healed from the traumas that he has experienced over the past years. The refugee charity he belongs to continues to provide him with the support and therapeutic provision he requires as he starts to build up a greater emotional strength to continue with his ongoing maturational development. It enabled me to become aware of the depth of powerful traumas that refugee survivors have experienced during their journey from wartime destructive attacks where there is little compassion, and to arrive at a stage where they can start to find a new beginning for themselves. There are still painful and unbearable emotions that they require help with and support to work through, but the extent of their resilience and determination built up in surviving some of the most unbearable experiences is something to be truly valued and admired by others.

Even with the support that has received, Hamid is still struggling to accept his past, and to strengthen a new starting point in his life so that he can live in the present and not allow his past to defeat him and control his future. This is a feeling that has been shared by many young people at the Baobab Centre:

Accepting the past doesn't mean defeat. Tell yourself: The past is not going away but I will not miss this present moment as well. It's hard but try and live in the Now

(Ellison, 2022:27)

The third charity for refugee and asylum-seeking children and young people that I visited gave me the opportunity to meet with two youth ambassadors, both of whom had been refugees in the past. They recounted their personal experiences and explained how it was very difficult and painful for them, when they tried to help others to understand how they adapted to life in a different culture whilst struggling with feelings of emotional and physical isolation. They explained what it took for them to emerge as individuals with a stronger sense of self when they are trying to integrate into the culture of their new country after the traumas they had experienced during the whole process of transition from leaving their own home country to finding safety and settling in the UK. They said that their personal experiences helped them to work successfully as youth ambassadors. They saw their main role as that of helping and supporting asylum-seeking children and young people to understand the reality they are faced with as they try to establish themselves into their new life. They were able to share their experiences and help the young people to find ways of working through their fears and uncertainties whilst they are having to face the realities which are necessary if they are to integrate into their new country both practically and personally. The ambassadors shared with me both the positive aspects of their lives and the negative barriers that they faced when they were trying to make their way in their new country, and shared aspects including behaviours and customs, which were quite different from the country they had left. Their own insecurities and fears of not being accepted were great, both on a personal level because they were unknown to people, and the difficulty in building up trust and new friendships, but also because they were experiencing emotions of separation and loss, particularly because of what they had to leave behind them. However, each of the ambassadors I met with had fortunately experienced a feeling of being accepted and responded to positively by those who were providing for them on their arrival in the UK.

One ambassador came with his family to England after realising that they would not be able to return to their country after a brief period of living in a different country. Although it was painful for all of them to face and accept the reality of their situation, they were able to share their anxieties, uncertainties, and sadness with each other. Another ambassador came to England on her own but after being placed in one family which did not work out for her, she was placed with another family where the parents were able to take her in and give her the emotional security and provision of needs which she required to help her to integrate into society. This helped her to understand and accept the elements of the diversity of her new culture and adapt accordingly.

Both ambassadors are now settled, functioning well and in employment. Positive family experiences have helped them to become emotionally, professionally, and practically integrated within the system, adapting towards creating a new life for themselves. With both of the ambassadors, their experience of being initially seen as an unaccompanied asylum seeker before being given status as refugee who could apply for benefits in the UK, was complex and a period of extreme anxiety. They had to work through this alongside coping with emotions of loss and separation from their country and, in some cases, experiencing the pain of losing their own or members of their wider family. These experiences have given them the insight from which they can support other young asylum seekers and refugees to manage and work through their own transitions into a new life and culture. They and other youth ambassadors recognise that the long-term outcomes for them personally in their new country are positive, whilst some asylum-seeking children and young people experience compounded trauma from their childhoods. The outcome for these young people may not be so optimistic because of their own internal emotional reality, the negative way they feel about themselves, and their lack of resilience. This inevitably leaves them feeling extremely vulnerable when having to face a new and different environment, and where they do not have the emotional capacity to access opportunities for education and employment without the support of specialist charities.

Conclusion

This chapter has tried to highlight the depth of emotions experienced, both positive and negative, by asylum-seeking and refugee children and young people in their attempt to create a new life for themselves in a country that is different and far from their homeland. I have truly been inspired and emotionally moved meeting and listening to them share their stories with me. These young people have all been subjected to harrowing experiences, having to bear what, at times, they found completely unbearable in their journeys to find ways of reaching a new and completely different environment and culture, in which they could live in safety and thrive. They have had to manage complex bureaucracy and deal with the practical aspects of living independently, learning a new language, developing friendships, and ultimately finding a place to be themselves and develop a sense of emotional security and trust.

The three charities described spoke of their work with passion and sincerity and show the strength, commitment, and the extent of the work needed to help these children and young people to manage their transition to a new life, with confidence. This is not an easy task for anybody, but the teams were anxious to continue to develop their own insight and understanding about the task required, and to have a positive impact on the lives of these young people.

The poem that follows describes how painful it can be for these asylum-seeking and refugee children and young people to trust, and begin to speak of the fears that they have kept hidden throughout their journeys to safety. It is only at this point that they can start to develop a new starting point to the next phase of their lives, one in which they can find a strengthened sense of self and identity, and look to the future.

This is the morning she begins,
To talk about her life,
Her talk is made of fragments of fear.
She is blind-walking towards,
A truth made more bearable,
By the absence of nailing works of knowing.
Diana Cant (2022:8) *Mouth Organ*

Chapter 8

A stepping stone to the future

The role of schools

Francia Kinchington

This chapter explores the role that schools can have on the lives of vulnerable young children and examines what school leaders and governing bodies can do to ensure a safe and positive learning experience in which vulnerable young people can thrive and learn.

The role of school in the life of vulnerable children and young people

Although the book has examined the experiences of children and young people in a range of care settings and provision, there is an overarching system that applies to all children from the ages of 5–16, namely, that of the right to statutory education. Schools, whether mainstream, alternative school provision, or special, act as a stepping stone to the future, providing key life skills and an education that prepare young people for life, the world of work, and further and higher education. All schools will claim that they are child-centred and that inclusion, equality, and education for all children and young people lie at the heart of their school philosophy; however, as Ofsted inspection reports have shown, some are better than others. Inspired school leadership and committed and professional teaching have the capacity to beat the odds, even in the face of poverty and deprivation. Schools can provide a safe, stable, and supportive community which fosters trust and friendships, and provides a caring environment where children are able to develop and learn, in spite of early privation and trauma. For some children and young people, trauma, neglect, and privation may not be a past experience but one they live daily. These are young people who live 'beneath the radar' and have not come to the attention of social services; children who live impoverished lives; children who are neglected; or children who might be carers for parents and carry the responsibility for caring for younger siblings without respite. The potential of the school, its community, and individual teachers to support and provide a place of normality and turn young lives around, cannot be underestimated.

van der Kolk (2014:422) observes that:

> The greatest hope for traumatized, abused, and neglected children is to receive a good education in schools where they are seen and known, where they learn

DOI: 10.4324/9781003132882-11

to regulate themselves, and where they can develop a sense of agency. At their best, schools can function as islands of safety in a chaotic world. They can teach children how their bodies and brains work and how they can understand and deal with their emotions.

Given that children within the care system may only amount to fewer than ten children in any maintained primary or secondary school at one time, the issue of the child's visibility is of particular concern. If children are invisible, they cannot be supported and provided for, and critically, their individual needs cannot be met. Children may be invisible because of the perceived stigma of being in care and so do not want to tell their friends or teachers and to be singled out as being different or a victim. Headteachers and Special Educational Needs and/or Disabilities Coordinators (SENDCOs) will have knowledge of specific children within the care system in their school, but not generally share background and confidential details with teachers. Although teachers will be aware that particular children are in care, they may not understand how the child's past experiences and inner world impact on their outer world, behaviour, and learning. Most children in the care system have suffered unbearable trauma during their life and, as a consequence, have little sense of belonging or of being a person who matters, with little trust in others. As a result of the trauma and the difficulties they have endured, which is often accompanied by disrupted schooling and poor learning experiences, they develop a resistance to learning and find being made to learn or keep to rules difficult to achieve. This can be professionally demoralising and frustrating to teachers, who are confronted with a small number of children whose behaviour may be extremely challenging. Teachers may lack an understanding of the link between early trauma, anxiety, challenging behaviour, poor learner identity, and the capacity to learn in a classroom setting. Breakdowns in behaviour cannot be managed by confrontation and sanctions which only serve to escalate 'acting out' behaviours because they act to reinforce traumatic situations. Failure by teachers to respond to the psychological needs of these children and young people, and a lack of strategies for de-escalating erupting emotions prior to addressing their learning needs, reinforces poor learner identity and inevitably results in underachievement. Poor literacy, numeracy, and interpersonal skills are cumulative, and often coupled with a record of poor attendance and escalating acting out behaviours. Violence towards others and self-harm are risk factors that may, by default, drive the child towards gang affiliation in search of friendship and a sense of belonging and ultimately involvement in criminal activity.

Children and young people who live in stable, loving, and supportive families have a good start in life and are shown to have significant advantages over those who have experienced missing or early distorted attachments. They tend to do better at school, attend regularly, and form meaningful friendships. In contrast, those who did not have a good beginning and were overwhelmed by traumatic experiences which have left them with depression and anxiety, find it difficult to learn.

They are unable to take advantage of the experiences that school offers and find it difficult to make friends.

> They do not get better of their own accord. They go onto lead limited lives, underachieving at school, at risk of consuming drugs and alcohol, and finding themselves increasingly in social isolation, suffering repeated depressive episodes. If these children have symptoms of anxiety, their prognosis is all the more worrying'.
>
> (Trowell and Miles, 2011:34)

Disrupted education throughout early life, whether through erratic attendance, constantly changing schools, bullying, poor learner identity, and lack of access to education or teaching that cannot address the child's learning needs, all have a profound impact on self-esteem and adult identity and inevitably limit employment options. This is reflected in the Ministry of Justice statistics (2021) that show that 57% of adult prisoners taking initial assessments had literacy levels below those expected of an 11-year-old. The educational progression of this group of young people into further or higher education is poor (Ofsted, 2019b:13), showing that at the age of 17, only 49% were in some form of education (34% were in education, 15% in training or employment), with 27% not in employment, education, or training (NEET), and 24%, for whom no information was known. For 18-year-olds, 46% were known to be in education, 18% were in training or employment, but 30% were not in employment, education, or training, and there were 6% for whom no information was known.

Given this failure, the question is: what can schools do?

The guidance that follows is intended to enable schools to see themselves as inclusive centres of learning excellence where vulnerable children and young people, specifically, feel secure, safe, valued, and confident as learners.

There are six critical areas that school leaders and governing bodies need to address:

i A reappraisal of their school's philosophy and vision

A school's philosophy and vision statement should be evidenced in practice. Specifically, schools should ensure the creation of a nurturing environment that will support not only the groups of children within the wider care system explored in this book, but also all children, including those that may lie at the periphery of the care system. It should be acknowledged that the experiences of some children may not be so extreme that they come to the attention of social services, and so suffer unsupported in silence. The school should be able to articulate how the school's curriculum, the school's ethos, and the 'hidden' curriculum, characterised by the ethos and relationship between staff and children and the children themselves, and the educational experiences offered, enable children and young people to function at a creative, social, and academic level, feeling supported, listened to, cared for, and engaged. A school should be able to articulate the richness of what it offers children and young people including opportunities for self-expression, self-management, personal development, and achievement.

ii Policies and practice

Schools need to have a systematic process of monitoring all children who are vulnerable and potentially at risk and the capacity to assess the progress of these children. The Ofsted (2019b) education inspection framework (EIF) (292) requires that all schools should have a culture of safeguarding. This means they should have effective arrangements to:

- identify children, pupils, and students who may need early help, and who are at risk of harm or have been harmed. This can include, but is not limited to, neglect, abuse (including by their peers), grooming, or exploitation.
- secure the help that children, pupils, and students need, and if required, referring in a timely way to those who have the expertise to help.

To address this, contextual information should be held for all children on the school roll. This enables the school leadership team to categorise and address not only safeguarding issues, but also the potential risk of academic underachievement. A focus on the information held by the school for children within the care system will enable the school to monitor their progress in terms of academic, behavioural, attendance, and welfare markers. The categories held include whether the child has a child protection plan, is designated a child in need, or has a current education welfare file. Additionally, identifiers for home circumstances are recorded. These include IDACI indices (income deprivation affecting children index), looked-after children, post-looked-after children, adopted from care, special guardianship, and private fostering. A further indicator is that of truancy, in terms of both incidence and patterns, which not only has an impact on the child's learning and educational progress, but also makes them potentially vulnerable to external influences such as gang exploitation. These indicators are important in monitoring the academic progress of children, especially in the case of multiple categories of risk, and consequently the multiple barriers of learning experienced by the individual child, and critically in evaluating the impact of the provision put in place by the school on the holistic development of the child.

iii Review funding arrangements

Examine arrangements for Pupil Premium (for children eligible for free school meals across the education system) and Pupil Premium Plus funding (2022–2023) which is available for early years, primary, special, or secondary schools, looked-after children (LAC), or service children. Pupil Premium Plus (PPP) is additional funding given to schools or the local authority for pupils who are in care, or who have moved to permanence from care, for example, through adoption; left care under a Special Guardianship Order (SGO); are in local authority care in England; and have left care under a Child Arrangements Order (formerly a Residence Order).

Additionally, every state school in England is required to have a 'Designated Teacher for Previously Looked after Children' (DTLAC), normally the SENDCO, who should be the contact point for the Virtual Head (VSH) appointed by the local authority. Their specific responsibility is to manage and link in with schools on behalf of children who are in the care of the local authority. The VSH receives funding allocated to the local authority, rather than it going directly to the school, and will agree how Pupil Premium funding will be spent to meet the needs identified in the child's personal education plan (PEP).

Table 8.1 shows how PPP funding is used by the local authority via their designated Virtual School Head to support identified vulnerable children.

Table 8.1 Use of PPP funding by the VSH

Local Authority: In-School Support

Therapeutic input, such as play therapy, art therapy, equine therapy, cognitive behaviour therapy (CBT)

Speech and language support

Counselling (where there is not and will not be CAMHS involvement)

Provision of counsellors and mentors to support wellbeing of pupils to maintain good levels of attendance and promote effective learning

Emotional support and mentoring through the use of professional counsellors and volunteer mentors

Life coaching/mentoring

Targeting young people to increase enjoyment of reading with foster carer, as well as reading attainment and progress

1:1 tuition in an academic area

Preparing children and young people for transition

Private lessons, particularly where the child can gain accreditation, for example, music, dance, drama, singing

Purchase of equipment for the child's sole use to support learning or development of a skill, such as a study pad, laptop, musical instrument, sports equipment

Book purchases

Costs associated with undertaking the Duke of Edinburgh award

Dyslexia assessment

Contribution towards costly residential education school trips (if all other educational needs are being met)

Local authority: provision of specialist training

Training for the designated teacher for looked-after children (DTLAC)

Attachment and trauma awareness training

Attachment practitioner training

Training for Foster carers: metacognitive training to support thought processes required for developing the organisational skills, executive function, and problem-solving strategies of the young people for whom they care.

The aim is to ensure that the needs of children covered by this funding are detailed annually, targets are set based on base-line and diagnostic assessment, and children's progress is evaluated in relation to the targets set. In contrast to the local authority provision provided via the VSH, in-school focused provision may include breakfast clubs, homework support, and after-school activities; provision of literacy and numeracy mentors; introduction of part-time counselling staff to support individual children; and specific training of staff to develop skills which can then be used as a resource for the school. These specific resources may include managing challenging behaviours, developing specialist areas of expertise such as working with children with low self-esteem, poor learner identity, poor attendance records, poor social and interaction skills, and supporting children to counter bullying and to develop life skills such as resilience and confidence.

iv The classroom and school environment

School leaders, teachers, the school governing body, and the wider school community need to examine how the needs of individual pupils can be understood and responded to in the classroom setting. The Special Educational Needs Coordinator (SENDCo) has a specific role to play in ensuring an inclusive environment and that all staff follow the school's Special Educational Needs and Disability (SEND) code of practice (2015), ensuring that all children receive the education that they are entitled to, specifically in the case of children with an Education, Health and Care (EHC) plan. The Education, Health and Care Plan (EHCP) is a legally binding document outlining a child or young person's special educational, health, and social care needs and describes the extra support to be given and how their needs will be met. Addressing barriers to learning may involve calling in outside professionals such as an educational psychologist, specialist teaching assistants, and other professionals to support communication and interaction needs; cognition and learning needs; social, emotional, and mental health needs; and sensory and/or physical needs as required by SEND (2015).

It is critical that the classroom is a safe environment for these children and young people to ensure that they feel contained, that they do not feel bullied or undermined, and where their learning needs can be thought about and responded to effectively, in spite of any disruptive or aggressive behaviour they may present.

These children and young people find it hard to believe that they can learn from their teachers. They are overwhelmed by the pressure in the classroom, especially where they have poor functional literacy and numeracy and a poor learner identity, and are unable to keep up with the rest of the class. Inevitably, their response is to become disruptive and either self-exclude or as a consequence of their behaviour, to be excluded by the school. Although they may be directed to alternative provision such as pupil referral units, this does not constitute full-time education and the wider opportunities that this offers, and often reinforces poor learner identity. Understanding how teachers can address resistance to learning to provide appropriate support and encouragement, enabling the child in care to feel a part of their classroom experiences in the school setting, is central to providing the starting point to enjoying learning in the classroom. Strategies such as small group settings and the use of age-appropriate nurture groups in the classroom setting offer a positive way forward and a psychologically safe classroom. The importance of nurturing a sense of wellbeing for the children, the role of language and behaviour as communication, the development of interpersonal skills, and the importance of preparing for transitions are vital elements.

Transitions are inevitably stressful and, for some children and young people, even traumatic. Transitions and the changes that they bring, whether from nursery to reception, primary to secondary school, moving from year 11 (compulsory education phase) into post-16 education, or moving to another school, all signal changes in self-identity, physical development, and emotional insecurity. Transitions also add another layer of uncertainty for the child or young person where they are forced to reappraise themselves and their relationships, to move away from the familiar and to try to make sense of the future and the unknown. However, these are areas where schools have a great deal of experience and are able to prepare young people to develop the confidence to look forward.

v   Mental health and wellbeing

This area is of particular importance and comprises two key elements, that of the school's ethos, which permeates the whole of the school, and the Personal, Social, Health Education curriculum (PSHE). The school's ethos is critical, not only to children in care, but also to all children and staff, and is evident and reinforced through student-student, staff-student, and staff-staff relationships. A positive ethos is characterised by a culture of inclusion where young people and staff feel safe, affirmed as individuals, confident, feel listened to, trusted, and experience a sense of belonging and part of a community.

The Personal, Social, Health Education curriculum, of which Relationships and Sex Education (RSE) and Health Education are now compulsory (DfE, 2019), is a fundamental but often unrecognised part of the school curriculum, providing both information and a forum for exploring difficult topics. The topics covered, which include not only sex and relationship education but also mental wellbeing, staying safe on-line, healthy living, drug education, and financial education, have the potential to support and educate young people for adult life equipping them with a sound understanding of risk and with the knowledge and skills necessary to make safe and informed decisions. Although the curriculum is created and taught by teachers, the school may also call on specialist health and social care professionals to enrich the curriculum on offer.

A school that defines itself as a learning community that is caring, inclusive, and psychologically safe, free from bullying and where each child and adult are able to learn and develop to the best of their ability, is likely to be successful. In light of the amount of time children and young people spend in schools and the detailed assessment of their progress that takes place, the school is well positioned to recognise the impact of stress, anxiety, and mental health on learning. A caring school community ensures that the mental and physical health of children are placed at the forefront of the school's vision, recognising the impact this has not only on the self-esteem, achievement, and behaviour of its students, but also on the mental wellbeing and professional confidence of staff.

The survey of mental health of children and young people in care in England in 2020 and 2021 aged 11–18 (Wijedasa et al., 2022:6) reported that

> The prevalence of mental ill health in the population of children and young people in State care in England is high, with statistics indicating that around 50% of children and young people in care might have a diagnosable mental health condition (for example, depression, anxiety, conduct disorder) compared with 12%–17% of children and young people in the general population.

The long-term effect of mental ill-health in childhood includes low academic achievement, reduced productivity, adult mental ill-health, fractured relationships, and a poor quality of life. Additionally, unaddressed childhood mental ill-health impacts not only the short- and long-term health, wellbeing, socioeconomic trajectories, and family life of children and young people, but also the health and social care systems through its impact on mental health services, the cost of interventions, and pressure on the State benefits' systems.

vi Specialist staff training and development

This will enable school leaders, the SENDCO, teachers, and the school community to develop both knowledge and strategies to help work with the child's or young person's resistance to learning where this is rooted in poor learner identity, lack of confidence, and underlying anxiety. The creation of effective strategies for the management of behaviour, ensuring that classrooms have a clear focus on learning and achievement, will help both the child in developing their learner identity, and the teacher in raising their professional confidence. Importantly, the discussion will also address how teachers can manage their own anxieties which occur when working with this vulnerable group of children and young people and develop a deeper understanding as to how unintegrated children and young people can be helped to manage formal schooling without acting out destructively or self-destructively. The SENDCO provides a key role in enabling teachers to develop a deeper understanding about the potential therapeutic nature of a classroom setting, one that enables children and young people to value themselves and gain the confidence to focus on their learning and achievement.

Conclusions

Christine Bradley

The aim and challenge of this book have been to deepen and strengthen the reader's understanding of early trauma and how the experience can influence our ability to manage the ongoing challenges of day-to-day living. Most of us at some point in our lives have been through traumatic events which have left us with feelings of sadness, pain, and loss. However, because mainly we can hold onto both positive and good memories in our minds through having internalised a sense of self and of being a person in our own right, it is possible with support, to work through the painful and traumatic times we have encountered. So, the question has to be asked: what about those who have been constantly traumatised, physically, emotionally, psychologically, and practically, and how has this impacted on the quality of their day-to-day lives? The majority of children and young people who are in need of specialist care have experienced a lifetime of trauma, with little respite.

The impact of trauma on the child's maturational development can prevent them from becoming an individual who is more able to manage the demands of external reality, especially where they have created their own reality in order to survive what has become unbearable and unthinkable for them. Consequently, they can so easily experience the outside world as being there to attack and abuse, mirroring the majority of their experiences in the early part of their lives. This can result in them becoming destructive or self-destructive in their behaviour and give rise to severe and long-term mental health problems.

My many years of working with emotionally vulnerable and fragmented children and young people has taught me that it is the ability of workers to be able to live alongside and respond supportively to the panic, rage, and deep anxiety in those they are responsible for, which is crucial. The role of the worker is to help find and uncover the child or young person's new starting point for themselves in terms of their capacity to live with, and feel more comfortable in their day-to-day lived experiences, and develop a sense of self in themselves that they feel satisfied with. This is more likely to occur when workers have been able to reach the heart of the matter in their work with them. The task for workers can be difficult and complex if the long-term outcome is to become more positive for those for whom they are responsible.

DOI: 10.4324/9781003132882-12

Section 1 of the book has been written to help readers who are en route through to thinking about the enormity of the task for carers when they are helping traumatised children and young people to strengthen their own sense of self. Presenting them with vignettes introduces them to the main focus of thinking that workers need to learn about when their practice is engaged with children and young people who have been consumed with the effects of traumatic events which have become embedded in their inner world of emotions. Chapter 2 in Section 1 is focused on the use of Needs Led Assessment and Therapeutic Treatment Plan programmes as an introduction to the way forward when the task is focused on helping and responding to the internal world of traumatised children and young people.

I have moved the chapters that follow into Section 2, to exemplify key areas of working practice with children and young people, and to recognise that all have had to manage traumatic episodes in their lives and the complex reality that they have had to face.

Chapter 3 on residential care examines the complexities involved when developing a therapeutic culture in a residential environment which is engaged with the treatment and therapeutic practice for children and young people whose life experiences have often been deeply traumatising. Placements break down where workers are unable to manage attachment relationships, and unable to manage the panic, rage, and unthinkable anxiety which can emerge through the destructive and self-destructive behaviour of the children and young people. The intention of this chapter was to give a greater insight and understanding to workers who are engaged with traumatised children and young people in need of residential care. The following two chapters, 4 and 5, have dealt with the difficulties experienced for their new parent figures when seriously traumatised children are placed in foster homes or adoption. It is hard for caring foster or adoptive parents to understand that children who have been severely abused and traumatised during the earliest part of their developmental lives are not going to be able to recover through simply being a part of a loving family environment and easily adapt and fit in with what they are being offered. The emotions brought about by the pain and attack of the early traumas leave the children expecting the same to occur again. It is because the experiences remain so deeply buried in their minds that it takes insight and skilled work on the part of the parent figure, to help bring about change so that the child does not recreate such experiences. Without appropriate consultation and training opportunities offered to adoptive and foster parents, the complexities and pain of bearing what has been so unbearable for the child or young person in their life will be difficult to live with, and the placements in danger of breaking down. Chapters 6 and 7 move into two quite different areas of work with traumatised children and young people, both who have experienced deeply traumatising periods in their lives. Chapter 6 examines how young people whose early lives have been characterised by trauma, chaos, and the care system populate secure units or young offender institutions where the focus is on incarceration rather than therapeutic intervention to address the potential of recidivism and prison. Chapter 7 explores the experiences and impact of trauma experienced by lone refugee and asylum-seeking children and young people in their search for safety and stability in a country far from the one in which they were born. The final Chapter 8 looks at the role and potential influence of school on the lives of vulnerable children and young people and offers guidance to school leaders and governing bodies. Schools as learning communities who have an ethos of care and inclusion can make a dramatic difference to the lives of children and young people, enabling them to develop resilience, relationships, confidence, and a learner identity that will offer them positive opportunities for their future so that they do not remain defined by the trauma of their early experiences.

Importantly, the aim of this book is to help readers to reach an understanding that traumatised children and young people can, with support, work through the traumas of their original experiences. It is crucial that those responsible for them have the knowledge, insight, and patience, to help them to arrive at the next stage of their lives with a belief that there is a way forward for themselves which is worthwhile and meaningful, and that truly is reaching the heart of the matter in the work in which we are all involved.

References

Abdi, S.M. (2018) *Mental Health of Migrant Children*, London: Oxford Research Encyclopedia of Global Public Health.

Become: Charity for Children in Care and Young Care Leavers www.becomecharity.org.uk

Bowlby, J. (1969) *Attachment and Loss. Vol. 1: Attachment*, New York: Basic Books.

Bowlby, J. (1973) *Attachment and Loss. Vol. 2: Separation Anxiety and Anger*, New York, NY: Basic Books.

Blades, R., Hart, D., Lea, J. and Willmott, N. (2011) *Care – A Stepping Stone to Custody? The Views of Children in Care on the Links between Care, Offending and Custody*, London: Prison Reform Trust http://www.prisonreformtrust.org.uk

Bloom, S.L. (2003). Caring for the Caregiver: Avoiding and Treating Vicarious Traumatization. In A. Giardino, E. Datner and J. Asher (Eds.), *Sexual Assault, Victimization Across the Lifespan* (pp. 459–470), Maryland Heights, MO: GW Medical Publishing.

Bowyer, S. and Flood, S. (2014) *Risk-Taking Adolescents and Child Protection: Strategic Briefing*, Dartington: Research in Practice.

Bradley, C. with Kinchington, F. (2017) *The Inner World of Traumatized Children: An Attachment-Informed Model for Assessing Emotional Needs and Treatment*, London: Jessica Kingsley Pub.

Brewer-Smyth, K. and Koenig, H.G. (2014) Could Spirituality and Religion Promote Stress Resilience in Survivors of Childhood Trauma? *Issues in Mental Health Nursing*, 35, 251–256. DOI: 10.3109/01612840.2013.873101

Cambrian Care Group https://www.cambiangroup.com [accessed 08.03.2022]

Cant, D. (2021) *At Risk: B the Lives Some Children Lead*, Guildford: Dempsey and Windle.

Center on the Developing Child at Harvard University (2016) *From Best Practices to Breakthrough Impacts: A Science-Based Approach to Building a More Promising Future for Young Children and Families* http://www.developingchild.harvard.edu

Centre for Excellence in Therapeutic Care (2019) *Introduction to the Foundational Training Program in Intensive Therapeutic Care Manual for Managers and Supervisors*, Abbotsford: Australian Childhood Foundation with Southern Cross University (NSW).

Cooper, A. (2018). The Development of the Self through a Secure Attachment (Chapter 1). In C. Bradley with F. Kinchington (Eds.), *Revealing the Inner World of Traumatized Children and Young People*, pp. 38–57, London: JKP.

Crawley, H. and Lester, T. (2005) *No Place for a Child: Children in UK Immigration: Impacts, Alternatives and Safeguards*, London: Save the Children Fund.

Crook, F. (2020) Times Article *'Prisons are Grim and Prisons Policy Even Grimmer'* https://www.thetimes.co.uk/article/frances-crook-prisons-are-grim-and-prisons-policy-even-grimmer-nv9hskl6r [accessed 10.09.2020]

De Bellis, M.D. and Zisk, A. (2014) The Biological Effects of Childhood Trauma, *Child Adolescent Psychiatric Clinics North America*, 23(2), 185–222.

Department for Education and Department of Health (2015) *Special Educational Needs and Disability Code of Practice: 0 to 25 Years* https://www.gov.uk/government/publications/send-code-of-practice-0-to-25 [accessed: 27.09.2022]

DfE. (2017) *Care of Unaccompanied Migrant Children and Child Victims of Modern Slavery Statutory Guidance for Local Authorities*, London: Department for Education.

DfE. (2019) *Changes to Personal, Social, Health and Economic (PSHE) and Relationships and Sex Education* (RSE), GOV.UK www.gov.uk [accessed 30.10.2022]

Diamond, J. (2017). Leading a Therapeutic Community, Chapter 2. In C. Bradley with F. Kinchington (Eds.), *The Inner World of Traumatized Children: An Attachment Informed Model for Assessing Emotional Needs and Treatment*, pp. 170–183, London: JKP.

Dockar-Drysdale, B. (1990) *The Provision of Primary Experience: Winnicottian Work with Children and Adolescents,* London: Free Association Books. ISBN 10-1853431028

Ellison, A. (2022) *Behind the Mask: Baobab Centre for Young Survivors in Exile*, London: Baobab Centre.

Felitti, V.J. (2010). Forward. In R.A. Lanius, E. Vermetten and C. Pain (Eds.), *The Impact of Early Life Trauma on Health and Disease: The Hidden Epidemic* (pp. xiii–xv), Cambridge: Cambridge University Press.

Felitti, V.J., Anda, R.F., Nordenberg, D., Williamson, D.F., Spitz, A.M. and Edwards, V. (1998) Relationship of Childhood Abuse and Household Dysfunction to Many of the Leading Causes of Death in Adults: The Adverse Childhood Experiences (ACE) Study, *American Journal of Preventive Medicine*, 14(4), 245–258.

Felitti, V.J., Anda, R.F., Nordenberg, D., Williamson, D.F., Spitz, A.M., Edwards, V., Koss, M.P. and Marks, J.S. (2019) REPRINT OF: Relationship of Childhood Abuse and Household Dysfunction to Many of the Leading Causes of Death in Adults: The Adverse Childhood Experiences (ACE) Study, *American Journal of Preventative Medicine*, 56(6), 774–786. DOI: 10.1016/j.amepre.2019.04.001. PMID: 31104722.

Fonagy, P. and Target, M. (2005) Bridging the Transmission Gap: An End to an Important Mystery of Attachment Research? *Attachment & Human Development*, 7, 333–343.

Foster Care Associates https://www.thefca.co.uk [accessed 08.03.2022]

Gao, M., Brännström, L. and Almquist, Y.B. (2017) Exposure to Out-of-Home Care in Childhood and Adult All-Cause Mortality: A Cohort Study, *International Journal of Epidemiology*, 46(3), 1010–1017. DOI: 10.1093/ije/dyw295.

Gooch, K. (2019) 'Kidulthood': Ethnography, Juvenile Prison Violence and the Transition from Boys to Men, *Criminology & Criminal Justice*, 19(1), 80–97.

Hart, D. and La Valle, I. (2016) *Local Authority Use of Secure Placements*, Research Report December 2016, London: DfE.

Hilder, L., Strang, H. and Kumar, S. (2021) Adverse Childhood Experiences (ACE) among Prolific Young Robbery Offenders in London: Targeting Treatment for Desistance? *Cambridge Journal of Evidence-Based Policing*, 1(5), 156–169.

HM YOI Report (2021) On an Unannounced Inspection of HMYOI CW by HM Chief Inspector of Prisons 9–13 August 2021.

Howe, D. (2011) *Attachment Across the Lifecourse: A Brief Introduction*, London: Red Globe Press.

Humphreys, K.L., Miron, M., McLaughlin, K.A., Sheridan, M.A., Nelson, C.A., Fox, N.A. and Zeanah, C.H. (2018) Foster Care Promotes Adaptive Functioning in Early Adolescence Among Children Who Experienced Severe, Early Deprivation, *Journal of Child Psychology and Psychiatry,* 59(7), 811–821.

Khan, L. (2016) *Missed Opportunities: A Review of Recent Evidence into Children and Young People's Mental Health,* Centre for Mental Health 2016 & Annual Report of the Chief Medical Officer 2012, Our Children Deserve Better: Prevention Pays.

Lewin, V. (2014) *The Twin in the Transference,* 2nd ed. London: Routledge.

McCrory, E.J., Gerin, M.I. and Viding, E. (2017) Annual Research Review: Childhood Maltreatment, Latent Vulnerability and the Shift to Preventative Psychiatry – The Contribution of Functional Brain Imaging, *Journal of Child Psychology and Psychiatry,* 58(4), 338–357. DOI: 10.1111/jcpp.12713

McMahon, L. (1992) *The Handbook of Play Therapy,* London: Routledge.

Ministry of Justice (2021) *Prison Education Statistics 2019–2020* https://www.gov.uk/government/statistics/prison-education-statistics-2019

Ministry of Justice and HM Prison and Probation Service (2020) *Findings of the Separation Taskforce: Separation of Children in Young Offender Institutions, Separation taskforce and Sir Alan Wood* https://www.gov.uk/government

Narey, M. and Owers, M. (2018) *Foster Care in England a Review for the Department for Education,* London: DfE www.gov.uk/government/news/independent-review-of-foster-care-in-england [accessed 06.06.2022]

Newlove-Delgado, T., Williams, T., Robertson, K., McManus, S., Sadler, K., Vizard, T., Cartwright, C., Mathews, F., Norman, S., Marcheselli, F. and Ford, T. (2021) *Mental Health of Children and Young People in England 2021 – Wave 2 Follow Up to the 2017 Survey,* London: Health and Social Care Information Centre, NHS.

NHCR, UNICEF and IOM (2019) *Refugee and Migrant Children in Europe Accompanied, Unaccompanied and Separated: Overview of Trends January to December 2019* www.unicef.org/eca/media/12671/file, https://displacement.iom.int/system/tdf/reports/UNHCRUNICEFIOM

Ofsted (2019a) *Children's Social Care in England, 2018-19* (Official Statistics).

Ofsted (2019b) *Education Inspection Framework (EIF),* Gov.UK https://www.gov.uk/government/publications/education-inspection-framework [accessed 06.09.2022]

Ofsted (2020) *Children's Social Care in England, 2020* (Official Statistics).

Phillips, A. (1988) *Winnicott,* London: Fontana.

Pieloch, K., Mccullough, M.B. and Marks, A.K. (2016) Resilience of Children with Refugee Statuses: A Research Review, *Canadian Psychology/Psychology Canadienne,* 57(4), 330–339. DOI: 10.1037/cap0000073

Pinto, C. (2019) Looked After and Adopted Children: Applying the Latest Science to Complex Biopsychosocial Formulations, *Adoption & Fostering,* 43(3), 294–309. DOI: 10.1177/0308575919856173

Prison Reform Trust (2016) *In Care, Out of Trouble. How the Life Chances of Children in Care can be Transformed by Protecting them from Unnecessary Involvement in the Criminal Justice System. Report of an Independent Review Chaired by Lord Laming,* London: Prison Reform Trust.

Radford, L., Corral, S., Bradley, C., Fisher, H., Bassett, C., Howat, N. and Collishaw, S. (2011) *Child Abuse and Neglect in the UK Today,* London: NSPCC.

Sadie, C., Holt, C., Harriott, A., D'Souza, S. and Watt, J. (2022). Children in Custody: Exploring the Impact of Incarceration for Children and their Families in the Context of

Wider Marginalization and Oppression (Chapter 5). In J. Tomlin and B. Völlm (Eds.), *Diversity and Marginalization in Forensic Mental Health*, pp. 11, New York: Routledge.

Schofield, G. (2005) The Voice of the Child in Family Placement Decision-Making: A Developmental Model, *Adoption and Fostering*, 29(1), 29–44.

Simkiss, D. (2012) Looked after children, Chapter 11, In *Annual Report of the Chief Medical Officer 2012*, Our Children Deserve Better: Prevention Pays, Department of Health. https://www.gov.uk/government/publications [accessed December 2022]

Sissay, L. (2020) My Name Is Why, Edinburgh: Canongate Books.

Taggart, D. (2018), *Trauma-Informed Approaches with Young People: Frontline Briefing*, Dartington: Research in Practice.

Taylor, C. (2016) *Review of the Youth Justice System in England and Wales*, London: Ministry of Justice, HMSO.

Trowell, J. (2002). Refugee Children and Abuse (Chapter 5). In R.K. Papadopoulos, *Therapeutic Care for Refugees: No Place like Home*, pp. 93–102, London: Karnak.

Trowell, J. and Miles, G. (Eds.), (2011) *Childhood Depression: A Place for Psychotherapy*, London: Karnac Books.

UNICEF (2019) *Refugee and Migrant Response in Europe Situation Report #34*, New York: UNICEF.

Vaccaro, G. and Lavick, J. (2008) Trauma: Frozen Moments, Frozen Lives, *Bulletin of Experimental Treatments for AIDS (BETA)*, 20(4), 31–41.

van der Kolk, B.A. (2014) *The Body Keeps the Score: Brain, Mind, and Body in the Healing of Trauma,* New York: Viking.

Wijedasa, D.N., Yoon, Y., Schmits, F., Harding, S. and Hahn, R. (2022) *A Survey of the Mental Health of Children and Young People in care in England in 2020 and 2021*, Bristol: University of Bristol.

Winnicott, D.W. (1958) The Capacity to Be Alone. In D.W. Winnicott (Ed.), *The Maturational Processes and the Facilitating Environment* (pp. 29–36), London: Karnac Books.

Winnicott, D.W. (1960). Ego Distortion in Terms of True and False Self. In D.W. Winnicott (Ed.), *The Maturational Processes and the Facilitating Environment Studies in the Theory of Emotional Development* (pp. 140–152), London: Karnac Books.

Winnicott, D.W. (1963) Dependence in Infant Care, in Child Care, and in the Psychoanalytic Setting, *The International Journal of Psychoanalysis*, 44(3), 339–344.

Winnicott, D.W. (1965) *The Family and Individual Development*, London: Tavistock Pub.

Winnicott, D.W. (1969) The Use of An Object, *International Journal of Psychoanalysis*, 50(4), 711–716.

Winnicott, D.W. (1971) *Playing and Reality*, London: Tavistock Pub.

Youth Justice Board (2015) *Keeping Children in Care out of Trouble: An Independent Review Chaired by Lord Laming Response by the Youth Justice Board for England and Wales to the Call for Views and Evidence*, London: Youth Justice Board.

Index

Note: **Bold** page numbers refer to tables; *italic* page numbers refer to figures.

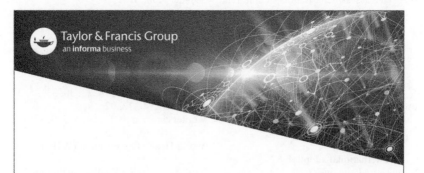